AcciDental Blow Up in Medicine:

Battle Plan for Your Life

Cancer, Lyme and Chronic Diseases

Simon Yu, MD

To Roger,

For Your Health,

Simon

AcciDental Blow Up in Medicine:

Battle Plan for Your Life

Cancer, Lyme and Chronic Diseases

1st Edition

This book is written for informational purposes and not intended as medical advice. The views in this book are those of the author, who has not been paid or sponsored by any institution for the content within.

Prevention and Healing, Inc.

For information, contact:

10908 Schuetz Road
St. Louis, Missouri 63146

www.preventionandhealing.com

ISBN 978-0-578-52417-7

Dedication

This book is dedicated to all of my patients who struggled to recover their health and stay well against the odds. Their quest and fighting spirit inspired me to search for the underlying causes of their illnesses. I celebrate those who have been successful on their journeys, and I have learned from all of them. Some succumbed to their illness despite our best efforts; their painful, disappointing experiences are not forgotten. They became a building block for the next successful outcome, which has helped lead to this book. Together, we are advancing on the knowns and unknowns of life, disease, treatment, recovery, and health.

Also by Simon Yu, MD

*Accidental Cure: Extraordinary Medicine for Extraordinary
Patients*

Reviews & Recommendations

"You hold in your hands the key to a healthier future.

If you want your *other* doctors to begin this journey as well, gift them a copy of Acci*Dental* Blow Up in Medicine and encourage them to study and learn from this exceptional physician."
John Trowbridge, MD, *The Yeast Connection*, Houston, TX

"In my wildest dreams, I could not have believed that I would ever have

gotten back to the place that I am today; I have literally gone from wrecked to recovered. I am truly blessed and forever grateful."
Scott Forsgren, *Better Health Guy*, Santa Clara, CA

"A true pioneer in our quest for health, Dr. Yu puts patients first.

He looks where few health professionals dare to look to find the causes of health problems: the oral cavity."
Douglas L. Cook, DDS, *Rescued by My Dentist,* Suring, WI

"Dr. Yu combines years of experience and expertise in Western and Eastern

Medicine, detailing his approach to chronic illnesses: a valuable resource for patients and physicians."
Carolyn McMakin, MA, DC, *The Resonance Effect*, Portland, OR

"All of this as seen through the eyes of a retired U. S. Army Colonel who looks at the challenge of chronic illness in the same way Sun Tzu's *The Art of War* addresses military theory and practice."
John L. Wilson, Jr., MD, Great Smokies Medical Center, NC

"I implore dentists to read this book and understand they have a choice to make. They can continue to be 'Tooth Carpenters' or embark on the most satisfying learning journey of their lives."
Blanche Grube, DMD, Centers for Healing, Scranton, PA

"Thanks, Dr. Yu, for enabling me to help poor village patients in India! AMA testing is a non-invasive and inexpensive test when compared to analysis of metabolic profile and hormonal assessment in functional medicine."
Vijay Mohan, MD, Divine Touch Clinic, India

"Encountering this book is an extraordinary happiness. It will be very helpful to doctors who want an advanced and comprehensive understanding of your approach to Medicine."
Wooryong Kim, MD, Seoul, Korea

Forward: For Patients

You are about to embark on a life-changing experience, totally expanding the ways in which you see how people get sick… and how to finally get better! Every day when you are suffering, you awaken with a fresh hope that today – *this* day – your doctors will help you begin to win the battle to restore your health.

Sadly, as the months and years go by, you fail to respond to usual medical care, painful inflammation worsens, and your hope falters as you realize you are *losing*. In this valuable book, Dr. Simon Yu, MD, opens up for you an entirely new vista, one where recovery is possible – by treating unsuspected infections and stealthy health problems, thereby rebalancing *energy* flows inside your body!

You do not have to understand electricity to know that plugging a device into an outlet allows it to function. You do not have to read Einstein to know that energy and matter are interrelated; you cannot have one without the other. You do not need to have any military experience to know that unless we understand the enemy, we cannot win, and a conventional military strategy may not be the way to win the war against an unconventional, asymmetric threat.

In the same way, an advanced form of biocybernetic energy evaluation – needle-free Acupuncture Meridian Assessment (AMA) – enables Dr. Simon Yu to go through the steps of detecting, treating and removing biochemical and bioelectrical blockages through a spectrum of conventional and integrative medical treatments. The result is revitalized energy flows.

The same way electricity makes your computer or phone wake up and work, and you reboot it when a virus or malware infects its software, each of your organs and systems that is no longer functioning well can be "rebooted" and restored toward normal. As your immune system recovers, persistent infections, heavy metals and toxins, inflammation, and even some cancers can come under control, symptoms can improve, and better health can be restored – often after years of "mystery symptoms" and declining health.

You've been to many doctors; they've looked at your complaints. You've been to dentists; they've filled cavities, performed root canals, and adjusted your bite. Likely no one has told you that many of our modern degenerative illnesses (and infections) begin just behind our lips, right under our noses! The Acci*Dental* approach to healing is comprehensive and includes unmasking and removing sources of infections and toxins hidden in your teeth and jaws. Dr. Yu can help pinpoint problem areas with AMA testing – and he can help confirm when your treatments are working.

This easy-to-read book will give you a working knowledge of the severe threats we face from fungal and parasitic infections. These are not Third World problems: these microbial assaults happen right here, every day, to every one of us. To do battle against these challenges to your survival (and the causes of your illnesses), you will learn lifestyle changes to strengthen your defense system. You might be hesitant… so you need to know that many people succeed, often more easily than they expected, thanks to the guiding hand of a caring and competent physician who has blazed a trail that others have never considered.

If you want your doctors to begin this journey as well, gift them a copy of Acci*Dental* Blow Up in Medicine and encourage them to learn from this exceptional physician. You hold in your hands the keys to a brighter, healthier future for you and your family.

John Parks Trowbridge, MD, FACAM
Life Celebrating Health, Houston, Texas

Onward: For Physicians

I've been treating patients for decades. All too often, success in treating patients leads to a casual conclusion that what you're doing is enough, *it's working*. For patients who fail to respond, we try other treatments or simply refer them to another physician.

But wait! – Those whose illnesses are difficult to treat... *those* are the ones from whom we can learn more about the hidden causes of disease. *Those* are the ones who should capture our full measure of attention – not a casual send-off. Simon Yu, MD has devoted his life's work and studies to discovering and addressing the deeper roots of so-called "undiagnosed" and "untreatable" human misery.

Hundreds of new patients each year find effective solutions to their health challenges through his guiding hand. Many more can be reached if more physicians, like us, broaden our horizons beyond our medical school training and routine conferences, and learn how to develop new battle plans to detect and combat asymmetric threats to restore normal energy flows and healthy metabolic functioning in the body.

As physicians, we are trained to look, listen, feel. But all too often, we are looking mostly at lab tests or x-ray reports. You might be one of the many physicians who have said, "Your tests all look fine, we're not sure why you're complaining." Scans and x-rays are supposed to look deep inside... but what if they fail to show "something?" Looking at a patient's teeth might only show a filling or crown here or there... but what if body-threatening infection is festering quietly, deep within? Gums and jaws are even more puzzling, since we ignore most problems "unless it hurts."

You may be skeptical. You may be asking, "If there is something to this, why haven't I heard of it before? Where is the medical literature? Where are the clinical trials studies? Where are the guidelines?" In our medical training, we physicians learn a rigorous approach, a style of thinking.

Like you and me, Dr. Simon Yu learned the rigors of medicine. Then, during his military assignments as a U.S. Army Reserve Medical Corps officer, he began to have uniquely different experiences than his work as the medical director of a Midwest regional health maintenance organization (HMO). He wrote many patients prescriptions to alleviate symptoms, but they did not improve from chronic illnesses. Through careful observations – and moving onward to study other systems of medicine, such as acupuncture at Stanford and German Biological Medicine at Medicine Week in Baden-Baden – he found he could help patients in ways he had never dreamed before. Rather than settling for these first realizations, he began to build upon them, gradually enlarging the number of mystery conditions that he could improve through systematic detection and treatment.

Many patients come to see Dr. Yu with serious, progressive illnesses, cancers, persistent Lyme, suspicions of parasites, and unexplained mystery symptoms. Others come with vague complaints of fatigue, generalized pain, poor sleep, loss of memory, and so on. *Where* should a doctor look to find a cause, a treatable problem to improve *these* conditions "when all the tests are normal?" Could their symptoms result from unseen, asymmetric threats, such as invisible fungal or parasite infections, hidden dental infections or dental materials reactivity, nutritional deficiencies, toxic chemicals or heavy metals, unresolved stress, bacterial or viral attacks, or lurking disturbances such as cancer?

Any one or several of these could be involved – so *which* is it and *how* to treat? We're familiar with printed lab results of cultures and blood tests and x-rays, allowing us to give marching orders, to go forth to do battle. But what about the modern stealth guerilla warfare threats to health? Those unseen, unsuspected and untested assaults which are responsible for *most* of our patients' suffering? This book will open you to another operating theater in which to detect the root causes of perplexing medical problems and treat them with greater success.

John Parks Trowbridge, MD, FACAM
Life Celebrating Health, Houston, Texas
https://healthchoicesnow.com/, 1-800-FIX-PAIN
Past President, International Academy of Biological Dentistry and
        Medicine (IABDM)
Past President, International College of Integrative Medicine
Author, *The Yeast Syndrome*, with Morton Walker, DPM

Outward: For Dentists

Dr. Simon Yu provides a roadmap for taking advantage of science to measure subtle electromagnetic currents to give us incredibly accurate information about the state of the body. Through Acupuncture Meridian Assessment (AMA), he can see the devastating effects of metal in the mouth. He can detect how infections in the soft tissues, around the apex of teeth, and inside the jawbones – called cavitations – deplete the energy of the body.

Dentistry is a noble profession but has created several generations of people suffering needlessly from ailments created by the very dentistry that was supposed to make them healthier. How do I know this? Read my story in Chapter 6…

I implore dentists to read this book and understand that they have a choice to make. They can continue to be "Tooth Carpenters" or they can embark on the most satisfying learning journey of their lives by becoming a real doctor of the head and neck. They can spend their day inserting toxic fillings, metal implants, and crowns, or they can learn how to remove those toxic materials safely and replace them with biocompatible alternatives, address hidden dental, gum and jaw infections, and work as a team of dentists and physicians to help patients regain their health.

Blanche D. Grube, DMD, FIAOMT
Centers for Healing, Scranton, Pennsylvania
http://drblanchegrube.com, 570-309-6198
CEO, Biocomp Laboratories, DNA Connexions, and Huggins
Applied Healing in Colorado Springs
Past President and active member, International Academy of
Biological Dentistry and Medicine (IABDM)

Preface: From Accidental Cure to AcciDental Blow Up in Medicine

Think differently!

All physicians are highly educated and trained how to diagnose patients' problems, treat them, help them feel better and restore their health: a high goal, a worthy challenge, and a lifelong professional quest. At least, that was my own expectation. Yet over time, I came to see that something was not right with our medical profession. I have heard too many times:

"My doctor said everything is fine! Why do I feel so bad?"

Warning: Your medical problems may not be what you think, what you have been told, or what has been diagnosed. This is the message of my first book, *Accidental Cure: Extraordinary Medicine for Extraordinary Patients*. "Modern" medical and dental treatments almost never deal with why these problems exist, while they frequently create new problems and side effects. We must address the *underlying* problems.

What, specifically, causes chronic illness? How can we discover root causes, which are often multiple and overlapping? How do they impact healthy functioning? How can we fix the underlying challenges in the body and restore health?

Patients come to me when conventional medicine has stopped working for them, and they see its limits. They don't want to give up hope. They want to investigate further, deeper, and consider new approaches. They want to uncover the causes of their health problems, rebuild their health and empower their futures.

Key to finding underlying causes and connecting the dots for patients is a new paradigm: Acupuncture Meridian Assessment

(AMA). This adds a new dimension and provides a tool to enrich and guide diagnosis and selection of treatments for patients. Acupuncture Meridian Assessment grows out of the history of ancient Energy Medicine, and it provides an advancing bridge between Eastern and Western Medicine.

> "Eastern philosophy looks at the human body as a microcosm of the universe. Western medical science dissects and analyzes the body as biomechanical and biochemical processes. It looks into the cellular and molecular levels but stops before going into the energy levels of the body. New research conducted by leading scientists from Germany is looking at the human body as a biocybernetic network of photon energy fields... What a beautiful concept if we can integrate these two fields of medicine!"
>
> Simon Yu, MD, in "Acupuncture and Acupuncture Meridian Assessment: Journey to East by West"

It is time to go into more depth on how to unmask deeper underlying medical problems and develop a "battle plan" to address asymmetric threats. This is essential to restore the ability to heal from challenging health threats such as cancer, persistent Lyme, and chronic mystery diseases. This book will focus particularly on how to use parasite medications and how to detect and refer for treatment of dental-related medical problems.

Functional and integrative medicine physicians have made good progress in recent years in addressing food allergies and sensitivities, nutrition, and heavy metals and toxins through chelation and detoxification. We are beginning to learn more about the interplay between genetics, exposures and epigenetics. Yet parasites, fungal and dental problems are still too often overlooked.

This book provides a resource for patients, physicians and dentists to sharpen and enhance their knowledge about parasites, fungal and dental-related medical problems. Patients can take this book to their primary care, functional or integrative physician (or biological dentist) and encourage them to explore these causative factors and get additional professional training in the field of energy medicine and Acupuncture Meridian Assessment.

My end goal is to encourage more physicians and dentists to get training and become familiar with these approaches so they are comfortable using them with patients. If we can correct hidden dental problems, parasite and fungal infections, and environmental toxins, a series of accidental cures may occur, and create an AcciDental Blow Up in Medicine as we know it.

This is important, given all the challenges we face: 1) hidden invaders: parasites, mold/mycotoxins, viruses, bacteria, and other infections; 2) the environment: heavy metals, toxins and pollutants; 3) what we ingest: food and beverage products, food additives and GMOs; 4) pharmaceuticals and medical/dental devices that can cause side effects as well as benefits; 5) accidents and physical and emotional trauma; and 6) sedentary lifestyles in a wirelessly connected digital world and widely interconnected physical world.

An Important Disclaimer

I do not claim to cure my patients, and never promise a cure. Healing and recovery is something the patient undertakes – physically, emotionally, and spiritually. My work is to remove obstacles to healing – to identify and address the hidden invaders – so that the biological terrain improves, making it easier to heal.

I am not an oncologist, and I do not treat cancer. However, I do see cancer patients and help treat their underlying problems. They come to see me for a second opinion and to look for nutritional support and immune-enhancing therapy. I leave chemotherapy to their oncologists.

I am not a parasitologist. However, I see patients who have parasite problems, and I have developed experience in treating them since my tour as a U.S. Army Reserve medical officer in Bolivia in 2001. We treated thousands of patients with antiparasitics and saw them report resolving a host of other medical problems. Parasites are not simply a Third World problem or an issue for people with animals or pets. Parasites and fungi often co-occur. Heavy metals and toxins can help fuel their growth and complicate treatment.

I am not a dentist. However, I understand the integral connections between oral and whole body health. I often refer people to see a biological dentist or oral surgeon as part of their healing journey. My initial patient exam will include looking for dental-related medical problems. I also test patients' teeth and jaws energetically to unmask problems that may not show on x-ray in order to assess their systemic impacts on health.

How do you detect these hidden problems beyond Western medical science based on blood chemistry, immune assay, DNA genetic testing, CT scan, PET scan, MRI, x-ray, EEG, etc.? Within the framework of biocybernetics, the tools of Acupuncture Meridian Assessment can be applied to detect and help guide treatment of root causes of underlying chronic diseases.

Embark on your journey, build your team, develop needed tools, and craft a battle plan to treat underlying causes and restore health.

Table of Contents

List of Figures

List of Tables

Introduction

This book shares new information, innovative approaches, case studies and experience, and doctor-patient journeys to illustrate what you can do to take responsibility to get to the roots of your health challenges and empower your health. It contains guidance for physicians, dentists, and other members of healthcare teams who work with patients facing serious chronic and "unexplained illnesses." For patients, it also includes practical health advice and tips that you can use to find new practitioners to work with to strengthen your "biological terrain" and improve your health.

I wrote this book in a story-telling format, my favorite. Start by reading Chapters 1 and 2 on the journey and quest for health, and how to develop a battle plan for your life. Read Chapters 3 and 4 if you need an introduction or review of the foundation concepts of my first book: Acupuncture Meridian Assessment (AMA) and Biological Terrain. Then, delve into topics of interest to you – and begin to envision writing your own story…

Part 1, **The Battle Plan for Your Life** introduces the concept of combining the patient's quest for recovery with a battle plan to counter asymmetric threats to health. Chapters include:

The Journey and Quest for Health
Develop a Battle Plan against Asymmetric Threats

Part 2, **Acupuncture Meridian Assessment: Key Concepts** recaps the introductory sections of my first book, *Accidental Cure,* and includes a new chapter on medical Acupuncture Meridian Assessment in action.

Chapters include:

Accidental Cure and Acupuncture Meridian Assessment
Biological Terrain and Biocybernetic Medicine
Medical Acupuncture Meridian Assessment in Action

Part 3, **Hidden Invaders: Dental, Fungal and Parasite Conundrum** focuses on the three most commonly overlooked causes of cancer and chronic diseases. Chapters include:

Murder by Dentists: A Mouthful of Forensic Evidence
Parasites as Masters of Deception
Fungal Invaders

Part 4, **Contesting Cancer, Lyme and Chronic Diseases** examines the three major health challenges that bring patients to Prevention and Healing for treatment. Chapters include:

Cancer: What Are We Missing?
Lyme and Persistent Lyme
Extraordinary Patients and Unexplained Diseases

Part 5, **Parasite Medication Guidelines for Physicians**, covers the decision-making process in prescribing parasite medications, common antiparasitic medications, guidelines and frequently asked questions, and detailed charts on parasite medications.

Parasite Medication Guidelines: for Physicians, Medical Hackers and Braves

Part 6, **For Patients**, includes health tips for patients with limited resources, recommendations for detoxification based on lab results, a note on self-help resources on the web, and information on how to find a biological dentist.

For Patients: Self-Help Strategies and Resources

The **Conclusion**, "From Accidental Cure to AcciDental Blow Up: New Medicine based on Acupuncture Meridian Assessment," calls for enlisting doctors, dentists and patients to learn how to develop battle plans to fight underlying causes of disease to restore health.

We all need to work together to fight cancer, Lyme and chronic diseases. I invite you to join me on the journey and quest for health, and develop a battle plan for your life!

Part 1
Battle Plan for Your Life

Chapter 1 The Journey and Quest for Health

*The journey of healing that you embark
upon – when you seek, find, and set a new
course, a new route forward – is your story.
You will need two essential elements
to begin this challenge.*

Have you ever wondered why you got sick, why your medical doctors did not know why, and what is wrong with you? What would you do differently if you found out that persistent Lyme, and certain cancers, were caused by unrecognized hidden parasites, fungal infections, and/or dental-related problems?

When you have medically unexplained symptoms (MUS), when you have been treated for Lyme and co-infections with aggressive antibiotic therapy or cancer with chemotherapy and radiation, and you are still facing chronic illness, persistent Lyme symptoms or a recurrence of cancer, you cannot expect to win with a different combination of the latest antibiotics or chemotherapies. In other words, you can't keep doing the same thing and expecting different results. Think differently!

An understanding of ancient Energy Medicine, based on acupuncture meridians – updated to the digital and quantum world – gives new insights and opens up a new dimension, another lens, for detecting causes of chronic illnesses. When all else fails, it can help enable physicians and dentists to connect the dots to make sense of missing information and links.

The Microbiome, Parasites and Biological Terrain

These major unappreciated problems – parasites, fungi, and dental problems – may plant seeds of deception for the development of cancer, heart disease or weird unexplainable autoimmune, digestive, metabolic or neurologic disorders. How? They wreak havoc on your microbiome and biological terrain.

The microbiome – many different forms of bacteria within us – is a popular new term to explain gene transfer, metabolism, evolution, and co-creation of the human species. The microbiome is the key part of your "gut terrain" that enables you to digest food and convert it to energy to feed your cells and body. These gut bacteria synthesize neurotransmitters, modify your metabolism, help clear waste and toxins through the lymph and organs of elimination, and much more – including your "gut feelings."

Parasites, fungi, and dental-related problems are the major unrecognized hidden disruptors of your biological terrain. Parasites are not a part of your microbiome but an advanced life form, classified in the kingdom of Animal, living in your body without permission. Parasites are unwanted, sneaky and potentially dangerous alien guests. Fungi are in a separate kingdom, distinct from animals, plants, bacteria, and more. "Parasitic relationships" among microbiome species is a separate topic.

Five Principal Causes of Chronic Diseases

What is the connection between these invaders of the microbiome and biological terrain, and chronic diseases and cancers? My five strategies for treating root causes of chronic diseases include:

- Parasite and fungal elimination with natural and prescribed medications

- Detoxification, including removal of mercury dental amalgam and heavy metals, chemicals, herbicides, pesticides, glyphosate, etc.
- Detecting and eradicating hidden dental infections
- Resolution of food allergies and sensitivities, and environmental allergies and exposures
- Nutritional and dietary support

The paradigm is rapidly shifting. Most integrative and functional medicine physicians have a good understanding of the importance of detoxification of heavy metals with chelation therapy, the food allergy rotation diet, and nutritional-dietary support. However, when it comes to parasites and fungal and dental-related problems, it is a "lost cause" for most patients and physicians. There are no reliable labs to test for them, and doctors and dentists lack training to detect hidden dental-medical problems beyond dental x-rays.

Dental Problems Can Be Dangerous, Even Deadly

Dental problems are considered separate from current medical conditions; some dental infections and reactivity can be hard to detect yet cause systemic harm. There are no reliable tests available to detect parasites based on current medical technology.

As people with pets – and veterinarians – know better than physicians, dental problems can lead to systemic infections, systemic inflammation, pain, growing dysfunction and other systemic disease effects. Too often undiagnosed, if left untreated, these stealthy problems are dangerous, and even deadly.

Sending the patient back to their regular dentist may not the best solution, since the dentist may have made the medical condition worse with root canals, amalgams, implants, and/or unnecessary wisdom teeth extraction which may lead to a cavitation or jaw infection. Redoing the same medical tests at different labs will be frustrating and fruitless.

Dental is the most difficult and often most expensive part of medical care, and therefore ignored by many. The financial burden of undoing dental-related medical problems without any guarantees of success is the number one reason why patients drop out. Delaying, dodging, skipping proper biological dental care may undo all your efforts and blow up on you. That is why my book is called, *AcciDental Blow Up in Medicine*. Don't be a slacker or stick your head in the sand about the vital importance of dental. How do you escape from accident-prone medicine and dentistry?

Acupuncture Meridian Assessment: New Forensic Science

What is an asymmetric threat? In short, an asymmetric threat refers to an unequal balance or an unfair advantage to the perpetrator, and is used in unconventional warfare. An asymmetric threat is one that occurs in an obscure, unusual or atypical fashion, and comes from a source that is weaker than its target. Asymmetric threats can be broad and unpredictable. They typically target weaknesses and vulnerabilities in larger and stronger organizations (or organisms).

How can we detect the asymmetric threats that are hiding inside - impacting your biological terrain, microbiome, metabolism, organs, nervous system, and more? When all else fails and you are still not well, and perhaps getting worse, it is time to consider Acupuncture Meridian Assessment (AMA). AMA can be used to uncover "unknown unknowns" such as parasites, fungi and dental-related problems.

Cancer and persistent Lyme are engaged in unconventional asymmetric warfare. We cannot counter with conventional warfare and expect to win. We must counter-engage with "unconventional technology" – Acupuncture Meridian Assessment, a form of biocybernetics – to disrupt, neutralize the enemy, and prevail against its asymmetric threats.

Think of Acupuncture Meridian Assessment as a form of biocybernetic forensics. Forensic evidence is that which provides evidence of a crime, theft, kidnapping, or felony. Chronic diseases and cancers are crimes against the body, biological terrain, microbiome, and/or metabolic processes. They rob, steal and kidnap health, healthy functioning, and the power of the immune system to restore health. If we can detect the crime – using evidence – we can work to combat it, through unconventional warfare, using the intelligence we gather through AMA to counter asymmetric threats.

The Journey: Quest for Health and Battle Plan

Fighting cancer and chronic diseases – a monumental challenge – can sap every part of your energy, family, finances, work, strength and enjoyment of life. The journey of healing that you embark upon – when you seek, find, and set a new course - a new route forward - is your story. You will need two essential elements to begin this challenge.

First, you need a quest: **the will** to keep searching for reasons, for promising and effective strategies, a will to do what it takes to get better and to never give up. This quest is your story. It will help define your journey and help keep you on the path. It will also help you connect and share with others on similar journeys, and to support each other, so your will, your quest, must be strong. You will need to feed your spiritual and inner compass and the light within you to maintain and strengthen and sustain your quest. This is vital and essential to strive for – to live for – to resolve to conquer your disease and regain as very best you can your health, vitality, and enjoyment of life.

Second, you need a **battle plan**. Not just any battle plan, but one that is up to the task of the unconventional warfare in the body: confronting hidden, asymmetric threats. We will start with a little background. When you are fighting cancer, Lyme or unexplained illness, imagine that you are unintentionally stuck in the middle of a battlefield sponsored by special interest groups. You don't know why and how you got into this mess. You wonder how you got into this war when you have regular medical and dental checkups, eat organic whole foods, exercise, take nutritional supplements, and have a positive mental attitude in life. How can you fight back when you don't know who are your enemies? Who are your allies? What is your greatest source of strength?

This is your battle. It is time to think differently. Antibiotics and chemotherapy agents do not correct the underlying problems. Disturbance of the "biological terrain" by some of the many threats to your "microbiome" is the reason why you have developed cancer, Lyme, or other mysterious or unexplained chronic diseases. Aggressive usage of antibiotics for Lyme may lead to increased fungal invasion of the biological terrain, creating an additional gateway for the development of cancer or other health problems. It is time for new medicine based on new biology, to address the asymmetric threats to health.

Contesting Cancer

If you have been diagnosed with cancer or recurrent cancer, you need to prepare a battle plan quickly, building a team to fight cancer and advance your quest for recovery. Imagine that you have involuntarily joined the military service and you've been assigned to the medical battalion. You were told by the government that we have been engaged in the successful military campaign for the War on Cancer for the last 40 years. We need more able bodies fighting to end this military campaign by the next decade. Winning the War on Cancer with more advanced chemotherapy, radiation, gene therapy and smart bomb-immunotherapies are our slogans.

Cancer is engaged in unconventional asymmetric warfare, and we cannot engage with conventional weapons and expect to win. We must counter-engage in unconventional warfare by applying unconventional disruptive technologies to neutralize and counteract the enemy and its asymmetric threats.

What are the main asymmetric threats? Parasite infections, including fungal infections, fungal mycotoxins, and complex dental-related infections are recurrent problems I face every day with my cancer patients. Strengthening the immune system by combating these invaders helps us fight cancer.

My Patients' Journeys

Patients come to my clinic in search of its name: Prevention and Healing. Some of my patients are local, and some travel great distances, from across the United States and around the world. They face a range of health challenges, from autoimmune conditions to cancers, cardiovascular, endocrine, gastrointestinal, respiratory, neurological and other diseases. The diagnostic and treatment process is a journey that we take together to discover and treat the underlying causes of their health problems.

Over the years, I have written more than 170 articles on a wide range of topics which are posted on my website; see articles page. You can also find many patient success and clinical case stories in addition to those included in this book. Note that I have changed many of the patient's names in the stories included in this book.

Ted's Story: Lung Cancer, Changing His Name to NED

Ted's journey has been so successful, he may change his name!

Four years ago I saw Ted, a 72-year-old retired banker from the Chicago area with stage 4 non-small cell lung cancer. I call him Chicago Bankster. He ignores my warped sense of humor. On a routine pre-surgery workup for a hernia operation, a CT scan showed multiple large lung masses and metastasis to his collar bone. He was not a surgical candidate. A University of Chicago medical oncologist recommended chemotherapy followed by radiation therapy, but his protective wife and daughter made a decision for him, outranking the Chicago Bankster: no chemotherapy or radiation.

Upon examination, his dominant problem was a hidden dental infection, along with fungal and parasite infections, based on Acupuncture Meridian Assessment (AMA). He started Clindamycin, doxycycline and itraconazole, and had seven bad teeth removed the following week by a local biological dentist in Chicago. It is rare that I can convince my patients to remove bad teeth on a first visit. It usually takes six months to a year and several visits to convince them why bad teeth must be removed. I tell my patients: no root canals or implants, and no argument with the dental recommendation.

Most stage 4 lung cancer patients are dead within six to 12 months. Ted was on multiple rounds of parasite medications, antifungal medications and insulin potentiation therapy (IPT, more on this in Chapter 9 on Cancer) to boost his immune system without using chemotherapy. Eighteen months later, he is stable, has been feeling well, and is active in his retirement, raising horses. Finally, a large tumor (4.6 x 2.5 x 2.1 cm) was resected, recommended by the University of Chicago oncologist. The pathology report showed a coccidioidomycosis fungal mass of the lung. He is still on fluconazole and itraconazole fungal medications, and you would never know he had stage 4 lung cancer.

Among the questions are: did he really have true lung cancer, or was it a fungal infection mimicking lung cancer? Or was it perhaps both? Were his dental infections related, separate and independent problems, or coincidental findings? Parasites, fungi, and dental infections are some of the most commonly overlooked underlying problems for almost all chronic illnesses. Other factors include diet, environmental toxins, heavy metals, nutritional deficiencies, and lack of understanding of whole body detoxification.

Since that time, four PET scans have been negative. His oncologist said there is no evidence of disease (NED), but is unwilling to say that he is cured. I also will not call him cancer free, but I agree that he is NED. Ted told me, "I am going to change my name from Ted to NED."

Fight Cancer and Invaders by Fortifying and Strengthening the Immune System

Our goal is to fight the cancer with minimum casualties in the battlefield. Right remedies in the wrong time sequence – without detoxification first – may set you further behind. You create your own success or failure, as beating cancer is essentially the ultimate war of the immune system. Everyone's immune system differs by genetics, history of exposures, and the interplay between genetics and epigenetics. Forget the statistics. Don't ask, "What is your success rate?" You are it. Family and friends may want to help you fight cancer, but they cannot fight for you.

This is your battle and your personal quest for health against cancer. You are fighting an insidious enemy. You may feel fine and the next month, you are told you have Stage 4 lung cancer with brain metastases or breast cancer with metastases to your bones. The enemy comes in many different shapes and forms. Your enemies may not be what you think, what you have been told or what has been diagnosed. Don't waste time or money if you are not ready to fight for yourself. You need a battle plan and understanding of the Principles of the War on Cancer.

If you look up the meaning of insidious, you will find it means gradual, subtle, stealthy and treacherous. Your objective is the same as mine: to identify, engage and defeat the enemy with minimum casualties. In order to succeed, you need directions on how to identify and engage the enemy, but the battle is on your own. To win the battles, you need to define your goal, objective, strategy, tactics and operation, and pursue them vigorously, with all you have got, as your quest.

Cheryl's Story: Multiple Myeloma - Whatever It Takes

Cheryl tells of her journey against unsurmountable odds, and her commitment to an ongoing, lifelong battle plan.

I am a stay-at-home mom in St. Louis with two daughters, both middle schoolers. My husband and I have a summer cottage in Michigan and spend lots of free time there, on the lake. In 2011, I was diagnosed with a malignant tumor in the area just above sinuses and soft palate.

At first, I thought it may have been an issue with my adenoids. I had contacted an ear, nose and throat (ENT) specialist two years earlier when I suddenly started having nose bleeds. He examined and scoped, saw nothing, and said I was getting older and had dry tissue so should sleep with a humidifier, which I did for two years. The bleeding continued, but the ENT never said to come back.

At age 45, I felt a lump in a lymph node in my neck, and went to the doctor. He called in the nurse. The next day I went for CT scan, and 3 days later an MRI. The doctor called on a Friday night, and didn't ask if I had time to talk. He said he was referring me to a doctor at Siteman Cancer Center. I had to leave five minutes later to get my daughter to a softball game. The next day I ran the school golf tournament, and then finally talked to my husband Saturday night.

On Monday, my doctor's office called and referred me to a head and neck surgical oncologist. He thought it was one of two types of cancer. I had a biopsy in 10 days, and learned it was neither of those two types. I was diagnosed with a plasmacytoma. Depending on the type, it can be much better or worse. If the tumor is contained, it is much better; with radiation treatment it will be fine. Otherwise it is much worse, and incurable.

A Biopsy Spread My Cancer: Multiple Myeloma, Radiation and Chemotherapy Options

My cancer was contained - until I had the biopsy, which spread it! I did 26 rounds of radiation on my head and neck, which was excruciating. I lost all function in my salivary glands, lost 40 pounds, and had no taste buds for a month after radiation. I had third degree burns on my head and neck. After waiting three months for the next scan, the news was not good. The cancer had spread to seven places in my body, and I was diagnosed with multiple myeloma.

The radiologist told me the treatment would be successful, but it was not. I was recommended to start chemotherapy, Revlimid. After the cancer had spread into my bones, he gave me five years and said I needed bone marrow transplants or chemotherapy; Velcade was another option. The nurse practitioner called and said,

"This is what you need to do." I was so sick from radiation that I wanted a second opinion. The nurse said, "Good luck with that."

My Path and Setback

I started seeing a chiropractor from my church who does a lot of Eastern type medicine, and I began doing a lot of research. My chiropractor said, "I think you need to start with Dr. Simon Yu." I began seeing Dr. Yu in July 2012.

I did everything Dr. Yu ever recommended: dental work including three oral surgeries to clean out two extracted wisdom tooth areas, parasite medication, detox homeopathy drops, supplements, hair analysis, and EDTA chelation. I grew up in Detroit which may have contributed to high lead levels, and a DMPS challenge test also showed high mercury levels. I had had my amalgams removed but had never had chelation before.

Food allergy testing showed I was highly allergic to peanuts, which often contain a mycotoxin, and soy, which is usually a GMO food, so I eliminated them from my diet. I also started ozone therapy mixed with my blood and recirculated, UV irradiation of blood, and IV vitamins and minerals.

I felt fine other than dealing with radiation fallout, until I fell snow skiing. Within five weeks, I broke my rib rolling over in bed. I developed a massive over-inflammatory response, which sent the cancer in my bone marrow into overdrive. After a CT and x-ray, a new doctor said, "I'm so sorry to tell you, you have cancer." My response: "No shit, Sherlock!"

They found several lesions. My immunoglobulin skyrocketed after I broke my rib. By April I raised the white flag and did Velcade shots for 8 months, two times per week. In the meantime, my right clavicle broke, my T6 vertebrae fractured, and my humerus in my left arm broke in half – simultaneously four broken bones. I had radiation in seven locations to help my bones heal.

The pain was beyond excruciating. Chemotherapy didn't help, but radiation mitigated the pain. Nothing was helping, neither Velcade nor vitamins/minerals. I said I was done with chemotherapy.

Insulin Potentiation Therapy

Dr. Yu had recommended insulin potentiation therapy (IPT) many times; I had rescheduled it, and I finally started. My baseline blood work showed a cancer marker, free kappa light chain, which was sky high when I started it. I did IPT weekly, and after three months, it dropped, and sixteen months later, it was much reduced, with all bones healed. I hoped I could go to every other week and then monthly. I started that but my numbers started to creep up, so I changed to the original formula and went back to once a week.

I feel fine, and am busy driving my children around. Within about two weeks, I had more energy and less pain. Dr. Yu says I am one of his "poster children" for IPT for cancer and other serious diseases. There are 12 ingredients, including antiparasitics, antivirals, antifungals, antibiotics, anti-inflammatory steroids, and some things to help the cells take it all in. IPT lowers blood sugar with insulin, so the cells are hungry. It also includes DMSO as a carrier, which helps kill the bad cells.

My cancer is in plasma cells in my bone marrow. It deteriorates bones from the inside out, so it is like blood and bone cancer at the same time. For me, IPT is a miracle, it is amazing. I don't know if it would have worked if I hadn't done the other things first. I also see a chiropractor, do daily coffee enemas, follow a ketogenic diet, do emotional talk therapy, Recall Healing, healing touch energy work, and acupuncture. As of now, my new oncologist doubts the previous diagnosis of plasmacytoma and multiple myeloma.

Persistent Lyme and Chronic Diseases

Those of you who do not have cancer, you can substitute your current diagnosis, such as persistent Lyme or Lyme associated complex, or other autoimmune, circulatory, digestive, heart, metabolic, neurological, or respiratory chronic diseases. These mysterious ailments of unexplained origins tax and vex you; they sap your energy, immune system and health, and lead to progressive breakdown of your body and its symphony of interconnected systems.

Unlike cancer, these enemies may be undetectable using conventional lab tests. They are stealth guerillas or hidden "sleeper cells" not known to medical authorities. This confounds physicians and patients alike. Under today's insurance-based medical system, no treatment, no medication is to be prescribed and paid for unless there is standard laboratory confirmation of the problem.

The challenge with Lyme disease and co-infections – when it is not diagnosed and treated appropriately up front, with a course of antibiotics sufficient to kill the Borrelia bacterium and any parasites that may have been transmitted, such as Babesia – is twofold. First, the lifecycle of the invading organisms gets established in the body. Second, additional problems and dysfunctions develop, which perpetuate chronic illness, even if the infections are eventually wiped out. You still may have chronic and debilitating illness. See my article in Chapter 10 on Lyme, "Who Else Committed the Crime of Post-Lyme?" Similar processes are at work in other chronic illnesses.

Given the nature and persistence of these asymmetric threats, as a patient you can do a lot to strengthen your biological terrain and immune system in your quest for health. But if that were enough, you would not likely be reading this book. We are talking about deeply embedded, hidden threats. You must seek allies to develop and execute the battle plan: a physician skilled at acupuncture meridian assessment (AMA), and a biological dentist and/or oral surgeon for any needed dental work. Other experienced health professionals can help round out your team and guide and support your journey toward recovery and wellness.

Jean's Story: Fibromyalgia and Mystery Symptoms

Jean says that looking back, she could have learned a lot about health from her childhood cat...

I first met Dr. Yu at an International Academy of Oral Medicine and Toxicology conference in 2012. Earlier that year, I learned from a functional medicine physician that my two decades of fibromyalgia and year of accelerating neurological "mystery symptoms" had been caused by a combination of dental mercury poisoning, persistent Lyme, and mold exposure from a week in a condo that had a major appliance flood that had not been remediated properly. I wanted to learn how this could happen – how we could still use a toxic dental material in the United States without informing patients of its composition or risk – and more about how patients can recover after years of exposure.

At the conference, I attended expert presentations and spoke to many people in the exhibit hall, including Dr. Simon Yu. I was intrigued to see a medical doctor attending a biological dentistry conference, and I bought a copy of his book, *Accidental Cure: Extraordinary Medicine for Extraordinary Patients*. It became the health book I most lent out to others in the years ahead as I met, shared stories, and networked with other chronic disease patients.

Working with a functional MD and biological dentist in my state, I made great progress in recovering my health, through removing exposed amalgams, getting better antibiotics to treat Lyme and co-infections, and working to clear my body of mold using Dr. Ritchie Shoemaker's protocol of testing and treatment. One of the biological dentists I saw recommended removing all my crowns and root-canal-treated teeth, as they may have had residual amalgam underneath the crowns, and there was evidence of infection associated with the root canals. He was an hour and a half away. Another, much closer, removed the exposed amalgams and treated me with a variety of antibiotics, which seemed to clear up the infections, but later they would return, and he would re-treat them. I was in a bit of a stalemate, as I felt great after the antibiotics worked, but the benefit did not seem permanent.

In 2016, I became a patient of Dr. Yu's. I was looking forward to him telling me to pull the trigger and have the crowns cleared and replaced, and my root-canal-treated teeth removed. During my first visit, about 13 out of 40 meridians were out of balance. It turned out my most pressing problems were parasites and fungi, which was not a total surprise, as I battled with parasites in the past. A month of antiparasitic and antifungal medications had great effect.

At the second visit, I learned I was ready to complete the dental revision and extract five root-canal-treated teeth. Although asymptomatic, many of them were visibly infected upon removal. In addition to using ozone and platelet rich fibrin (PRF), I needed additional rounds of antibiotics to clear the infections. This further improved my health, and I began oral chelation. At a subsequent visit, I learned there was still a cavitation problem in the lower jaw where a wisdom tooth had been removed in my teens; I had oral surgery to clean out that cavitation.

None of this was a surprise to me. I did not have a great immune system as a child, and I got frequent infections. I thought this might be why I got so many cavities and fillings in the first place, compared to my sister and brother, who had similar diets, but fewer cavities. I had experienced years of TMJ and mild jaw pain, which resolved when I took antibiotics for anaerobic infections, but recurred until my root-canal-treated teeth were removed.

Looking back, I could have learned a lot about health from my childhood cat, which died late in life of infections from tooth and gum disease. Teeth are markers of growth and development, and also of decline and ill health. They are like little land mines that can explode in the body. Treating pain with root canals is a bad solution, as it leaves dead tissue, which can become a breeding ground for bacteria, fungi, parasites and viruses. Teeth are God's plan for mortality, and Man's plan for morbidity. It is time to put them front and center in medicine and healthcare.

The Journey and Quest for Health

Many of my patients have been on incredible journeys, losing their health to unexplained illness, cancers, or serious chronic diseases, and not finding solutions in conventional medicine. They may have seen lots of doctors and specialists and tried scores of treatments and medications that may provide some help with symptoms, but often have troubling side effects. They are not well, but instead of giving up hope, they keep seeking.

Patients have so many sources of information today. In addition to doctors and all kinds of traditional and alternative books and articles on health conditions and treatments, there are also multimedia advertising pitches for promising (and expensive) new drugs, chronic disease associations, patient support groups, blogs, and social media. Social media helps connect patients – and practitioners – with similar interests, through blog sites, Facebook groups, webinars, Twitter and more. Patients share experiences and trade stories, ask for feedback and helpful referrals, and expand their horizons.

When conventional medicine lets you down and treatments are not working, when you are still sick and perhaps getting worse - you can either give up, or seek new approaches. You cannot keep doing the same thing and expecting different results. If fighting diseases with today's "treatments" is not working, how about finding the hidden, asymmetric threats that are triggering your disease through a forensic approach? Then, systematically work to eradicate these threats, and thereby restore your biological terrain, the foundation of health.

What is your story? What is your quest? What is your journey to date? Next, we turn to developing a battle plan to counter the asymmetric threats that are causing cancer, persistent Lyme, and chronic diseases.

Chapter 2 Develop a Battle Plan against Asymmetric Threats

My basic belief is that we should not fight symptoms,
a diagnosis or a syndrome, but correct the underlying
asymmetric threats.

Can you fight disease when you don't know who your enemies are? Familiar with Martial Arts and U.S. Army Military Medicine, it was quite natural for me to learn and embrace the concepts of biocybernetics and energy medicine that combine the wisdom of the Eastern philosophy with Western science and technology, and with the principles of the Art of War.

My basic belief is that we should not fight symptoms, a diagnosis or a syndrome, but correct the underlying asymmetric threats. By fixing problems in the biological terrain, biocybernetic matrix and microbiome, we let the body heal itself. In fact, I make an extra effort to ignore my patients' symptoms, diagnosis or syndrome, as these can be misleading.

Throughout this chapter, I will refer to modern U.S. Army military strategies combined with themes from military strategist Sun Tzu's book, *The Art of War.* Sun Tzu (544 B.C. - 496 B.C.) is considered the father of Eastern military strategy. His ancient Chinese book, *The Art of War,* has had a significant influence on Asian history and culture. In Western society, Sun Tzu's work has grown to influence modern warfare as well as politics, business, and sports.

Here is one of my favorite quotes:

"The supreme art of war is to subdue the enemy without fighting."

Know Your Enemy and the Art of War on Cancer

In the War on Cancer, we do not even know who our enemies are. One of the main tenets of *The Art of War* by Sun Tzu is know your enemy and know yourself:

"If you know the enemy and know yourself, you need not fear the results of a hundred battles. If you know yourself but not the enemy, for every victory gained you will also suffer a defeat. If you know neither the enemy nor yourself, you will succumb in every battle."

As I have explained, this book's theme is the planning and implementation of a military-style campaign against cancer and chronic disease, as we explore what works and what does not.

My goal in writing this second book is to formulate an effective strategy and battle plan for dealing with cancer, Lyme, or other chronic illnesses. I believe that you can replace the word "cancer," as in the War on Cancer, with almost any illness from which you are suffering. The War on Cancer can become the war on autism, Lyme, chronic fatigue, diabetes, fibromyalgia, lupus, heart disease, irritable bowel syndrome, migraines, multiple sclerosis, psychiatric problems, or numerous other diseases.

America's War on Cancer, declared by President Richard Nixon in 1971, was stymied or lost a long time ago. We pretend we are still fighting a successful war against cancer by painting a rosy picture of success rates and treating cancer patients like war heroes. The truth is, without an effective battle plan, too many cancer patients still bravely fight their disease, but then die either from the *treatment itself* or the *advance of the disease.*

I first presented my thoughts on applying military approaches to fighting cancer at a 2006 lecture during my Army Reserve mission at the U.S. Army Hospital at Landstul, Germany, where I was activated during operation *Enduring Freedom,*. My presentation was based on my military training and schooling from the basic and advanced officers' courses, and at the Command and General Staff College (CGSC) at Fort Leavenworth, Kansas.

CGSC is a graduate school for the United States Army, sister service officers, interagency representatives, and international military officers. The officers' course is a two year program. I completed half of the training as a Lieutenant Colonel, but did not complete the second half because of frequent calls to active duty.

In my lecture, I stated my objective: to apply my CGSC military training to medicine. I believe the principles of modern warfare can be applied in the medical arena by regarding cancer not through the lens of conventional warfare, but *unconventional warfare*. A key aspect of military strategy emphasizes the importance of asymmetric unconventional warfare.

From the perspective of modern medicine, asymmetric medical threats come from overlooking hidden dental problems and unrecognized infections, especially parasites and fungi, and from medical treatments weakening the immune system. Others include environmental toxicities, heavy metals, food allergies, genetically modified foods, and nutritionally depleted junk foods. One needs to focus on systematically identifying and eliminating asymmetric threats, which is more of a defensive strategy to rebuild the immune system and strengthen its ability to neutralize cancer.

As a retired Army Reserve officer, I read the *Army Times*, and one day I came across an unusual story about a lieutenant colonel who was urging the firing of unaccountable generals. Active duty Army officer Lieutenant Colonel Daniel L. Davis submitted a classified

86-page report to members of Congress in 2012 that documented the failings of U.S. policy in Afghanistan.

In addition, LTC Davis wrote an article published by the *Armed Forces Journal*, "Truth, Lies and Afghanistan: How Military Leaders Have Let U.S. Down."[1] He claimed that senior leaders of the Department of Defense, both uniformed and civilian, had intentionally and consistently misled the American people and Congress on the conduct and progress of the Afghan War. It was picked up by a wide range of publications.

Davis' essay helped motivate me to write a comparison of the art of war and the War on Cancer. Lieutenant Colonel Davis was fed up with "rosy official statements" that painted the war in Afghanistan as a picture of progress. He demanded military leaders come clean about the "absence of success on virtually every level."

The War on Cancer, declared by President Nixon in 1971, and renewed by successive directors of the National Institutes of Health's (NIH) National Cancer Institute, has been misguided and misinformed, and needs tremendous changes and a shake-up at the highest level.

Medicine's Offensive Strategy against Cancer

In military operations, to "go on the offensive" means to initiate an assault. In contrast, a defensive strategy is a wait-and-see approach, or reacting to an opponent's moves. The cell-kill approach to conquering cancer is an aggressive assault with chemotherapeutic agents that almost always involves radiation.

In current military thought, tactics are considered the lowest form of planning. Strategies are considered a higher form of planning. Strategic decisions are those that achieve the greatest value regardless of immediate return. There is a difference between winning the battle and winning the war, based on financial, political and military or medical strategies.

In military terms, tactics are techniques used to organize a military force to defeat an enemy. Military "tactical decisions" are those that are made to achieve the greatest immediate value.

In wars before the nineteenth century, military tactics were concerned with maneuvers on the battlefield. Today, military decisions are much more specialized, reflecting a need to deal with much more than the deployment of forces in the open. Operationally, modern military strategy includes asymmetric warfare, a new kind of battlefield where you do not always know who your enemies are.

Utilizing Asymmetric Strategies and Tactics

The word asymmetry refers to an absence of symmetry or lack of proportion between the parts of something. In his paper, "Defining Asymmetric Warfare," written for the Institute of Land Warfare for the United States Army, Major David L. Buffaloe quotes President John F. Kennedy, who provided this description of asymmetric warfare in his address to the West Point class of 1962:

"This is another type of war, new in its intensity, ancient in its origin — war by guerrillas, subversives, insurgents, assassins, war by ambush instead of by combat; by infiltration, instead of aggression, seeking victory by eroding and exhausting the enemy instead of engaging him... It preys on economic unrest and ethnic conflicts. It requires in those situations where we must counter it, and these are the kinds of challenges that will be before us in the next decade if freedom is to be saved, a whole new kind

*of strategy, a wholly different kind of force, and therefore a
new and wholly different kind of military training."* [2]

In his paper, Major Buffaloe explains that the concept of
asymmetric warfare has been around for centuries. Every time a
new tactic or invention changes the fortunes and power of one
army over another, an imbalance or asymmetry occurs, with
weighting to one side creating conditions for victory. Examples
include:

Greek Phalanx Formation

A formation in ancient Greek warfare consisting of a
rectangular mass of infantry armed with spears, pikes (10-25
foot long thrusting spear), or sarissas (11 to 21 foot spear).

Hannibal's Feint

Feints are maneuvers designed to distract or mislead, done by
giving the impression that a certain maneuver will take place,
while in fact another or even none will occur.

Genghis Kahn's Toumans

This example is from *The Art of Warfare on Land,* by David G.
Chandler. A touman is a Mongol military unit under Mongol
Genghis Khan (1162-1227) with 10,000 cavalry (warriors on
mounted horseback). Each horseman was an expert marksman
who carried his own weapons, tools, rations and clothing.
Highly mobile and deadly, Mongol warfare was complete
terror with superior mobile firepower, deceptions, and a global
intelligence system.

The asymmetric warriors I've described were much smaller but
more advanced than their opponents. In a battle with a powerful
conventional opponent, they might as well be invisible. They often

overwhelm a larger and less sophisticated military juggernaut due to the element of surprise.

Surprise, Denial and Deception: Ultimate Asymmetric Threats

At a May 2012 conference, "Countering Asymmetric Threats: A National Imperative," in Washington, D.C., keynote speakers Admiral James A. Winnefeld, Jr., Vice Chairman of the Joint Chiefs of Staff, and retired Air Force General Kevin P. Chilton, former Commander, U.S. Strategic Command, referred to surprise, denial and deception as the ultimate asymmetric threats.

In their remarks, they explained that surprise, denial and deception interfere with our ability to assess intentions, capabilities and other threats. They impede our ability to make timely and optimal decisions. Surprise, denial and deception are some of the oldest tricks in the book. Yet, history shows us these are tricks we fall for over and over again!

The speakers explained that because surprise, denial and deception are psychological phenomena, they cannot be prevented. Surprise, denial and deception are successful because they challenge the perceptions that fill the very **large gap** between what is **known and unknown.**

Recall former Defense Secretary Donald Rumsfeld's noted quote:

"The message is that there are no 'knowns.' There are things we know that we know. There are known unknowns. That is to say there are things that we now know we don't know. But there are also unknown unknowns. There are things we don't know we don't know."[3]

Observations and events are filtered through a prism of culture, assumptions, biases, and experiences. This leads military commanders – or in our case, medical professionals and/or patients – to mistake the unfamiliar with the improbable. This explains why collecting a vast amount of **Big Data** does not necessarily lead to better situational awareness and decision superiority.

Surprise, Denial and Deception in Healthcare

If the United States is engaged in a War on Cancer, what are examples of surprise, denial and deception?

Surprise

Measures designed to convince a cancer patient that he/she is a victim and that there is no known cause. The primary cause of cancer was discovered 70 years ago by Otto Warburg, PhD, MD, a German scientist who received the Nobel Prize.

Denial

There are inaccurate statistics concerning the prevalence of cancer. Denial of widely available and inexpensive natural remedies leaves the public with the narrow options of chemotherapy, radiation and surgery.

Deception/Diplomacy/Fake News

Various cancer awareness campaigns are working to convince the public that foundations and government and research organizations seek to find the fastest and best cures for cancer. These campaigns typically favor costly new patented, highly profitable therapies.

Hidden Enemies: Threats in the War Against Cancer

The list below introduces the hidden enemies that impact our biological terrain and health.

1) Parasites and Fungi

My first book explains my accidental discovery of a connection between parasites, chronic illnesses, and cancers. There are no reliable medical laboratory tests for parasites as they often live outside the GI tract, yet when these invaders are neutralized, cancer often disappears, or it at least stabilizes the patient's overall condition. Fungi also have a parasitic relationship with the human body, compromise its healthy functioning, and are synergistic in fueling cancer and other diseases. It can be said that parasites, not humans, are at the top of the food chain and exert control over human behavior and health, and fungi are our chief undertaker.

2) Dental Focal Infections

Focal infection refers to an infection in one part of the body that travels to, and creates an infection in, another part of the body. In the early 1900s, Weston Price, DDS, published research demonstrating that germs from a walled-off area (such as a root canal or cavitation resulting from an incompletely extracted tooth) can metastasize to other organs and tissues. He also demonstrated that putting such an infected tooth in an animal quickly led to disease. Dental infection has the propensity to settle in the joints, kidney, heart, and brain/nervous system.

3) Heavy Metals and Chelation Therapy

Metal accumulation in the body disrupts the body's metabolism and meridian system, setting up conditions for degenerative diseases such as cancer to occur. Heavy metals interfere with our metabolism by blocking the function of essential trace minerals, thereby damaging our immune system. Heavy metals make one more vulnerable to viral, bacterial, fungal and parasite infections. Almost all cancer patients have significant heavy metals exposure and burden that shows up using a provocation test with chelating agents. The most common heavy metals associated with cancer are mercury, lead, cadmium and nickel.

4) Malnutrition and Poor Eating (need for a Metabolic Diet)

The body has hundreds of metabolic pathways that require constituent nutrients obtained from food. Today's agricultural practices have depleted the soil of natural nutrients, making it difficult to obtain essential nutrients. In addition, the typical American diet includes far too many carbohydrates and sugars, and a host of food products and ingredients not well suited for proper digestion. There is increasing attention to the value of an individualized metabolic diet in managing cancer. Diet should be adapted to one's own metabolic pathways, which vary by rate of oxidation – slow oxidizer vs. fast oxidizer (measured by mineral ratios in hair analysis) – blood type and other factors, including food allergies and sensitivities.

5) GMOs

A genetically modified organism (GMO) is an organism whose genetic material has been altered using genetic engineering. Synthetic DNA is rejected by the body, causing deterioration and disease. Americans get less news about health risks of GMOs than in Europe, where GMO foods are carefully regulated by the European Food Safety Authority. The problems of "wheat belly," "corn butt," and "soybean heads" are accelerated by GMOs.

6) Allergies and Altered Autoimmune Response

The incidence of allergies is rising rapidly in developed countries. The growth in frequency and underlying problems is an indication of the broad spectrum of changes in body biochemistry. As microbiomes and gut linings are impacted, new allergies, autoimmune reactions and sensitivities develop. In addition to foods, personal care, household and yard products, pets, dust, molds and outdoor allergens, dental materials and other medical devices inserted into the body can have systemic allergic and autoimmune impacts. Patients should be screened in advance using a BioComp Labs or Clifford Labs test for dental materials, or a MELISA test and patch testing for medical device materials.

7) Environmental Toxins

Increasing pollution with environmental toxins helps lead to accumulation of toxic material in the body's liver ducts. Toxic overload creates a burden on the body's biliary tree, or network of ducts that branch through the liver and gallbladder. As noted above, installed medical and dental devices can be hidden environmental toxins under the skin and inside the mouth, hiding in plain sight, under our noses.

Environmentally sensitive people are the canaries in the coal mine, warning us of rapidly changing environmental toxic burdens in our bodies. Surprisingly, liver function tests often do not reveal the problems until they are far advanced. All cancer patients have liver problems. A gallbladder/liver flush (see instructions in Chapter 13) is an excellent supportive treatment, along with coffee enemas.

8) Trauma and Toxic Emotions

Physical and emotional trauma, from childhood to the present, takes its toll on patients' immune systems. Physical trauma can include motor vehicle accidents, falls, sports injuries, violence, and other injuries. Emotional trauma can result from illness, physical injuries, abuse and neglect, life setbacks, and loss of family members and loved ones. There is added emotional and financial stress of cancers and undiagnosed diseases, anger at lack of timely diagnosis, effective treatment by physicians and specialists, and adequate insurance coverage. Stress also comes from concern for financial and emotional impacts on family members and friends. These factors add additional stresses that must be countered, managed and alleviated to promote health.

9) HMOs and Health Insurance

A health maintenance organization (HMO) is a business that provides managed care for health insurance, self- or company-funded healthcare benefit plans, to individuals, companies, and other entities in the United States. Critics say that HMOs (particularly those run for profit) increase administrative costs and cherry-pick healthier patients. Health insurance plans also limit health care within changing government regulations.

10) Pharmaceutical, Devices and Health Product Companies

In 2016, global spending on prescription drugs topped $1.1 trillion, and it is expected to reach $1.5 trillion by 2021.[4] According to the Center for Responsive Politics' database, the pharmaceutical and health products industry spent $280 million in 2017, and $2.7 billion, on lobbying activities from 2007 to 2017, more than any other industry.[5] To ensure profits, drug companies persuade doctors that drugs are a solution for all diseases, including off-label uses.

Create Your Battle Plan for Health

You need to know some basic military lessons to create a battle plan for health. My intent is not to cover each subject in depth.

You can use the following list when I refer to tasks for you to perform to fight a War on Cancer, Lyme and chronic diseases.

- Know Your Enemy
- Know Yourself
- Know Your Terrain
- Asymmetric Threats
- The Law of War
- Rules of Engagement
- Medical/Legal/Economic Considerations
- Terrorism/Counter Terrorism
- Sabotage/Counter-Intelligence
- Collateral Damages and Friendly Fire
- Public Opinions/Civil Affairs
- Military Intelligence/Cyber Warfare
- Psy-Ops for psychological operation
- Special Operations and Black Ops
- War, Exit Strategy and Prevention of Next War

Management of Space, Time and Intelligence

The other important part of the battle plan includes *force management of space, time and intelligence:*

- **Area of Target**: Tumor
- **Area of Operation**: Whole Body
- **Battle Space**: Family, Job, HMO/Insurance, Home Environment
- **Time and Stage**: Beginning or end of last stage of disease phase.
- **Medical Intelligence**: Based on conventional and unconventional medical information.

Some of the principles may seem obvious—such as Know Your Enemy and Know Yourself. However, there may be more to these principles that are not as clear cut as they appear. I will not elaborate too extensively, since this book is designed as a simple survival guide with instructions on how to neutralize the enemy. However, some of these principles are worth exploring in-depth to prepare you to fight cancer. Throughout the book, I will cover these topics with a special emphasis on asymmetric threats.

Advanced Training on the Principles of War

Now that you have completed basic training, let's go through the checklist of topics you need to know from basic principles of war (aspects of warfare that are universally true and relevant). The topics in this chapter are part of lessons from the United States Army Command and General Staff College (CGSC) at Fort Leavenworth. I have used familiar military terms and analogies to explain concepts as simply as possible. I have also tried to apply the KISS principle first used by Kelly Johnson (1910-1990), lead aeronautical engineer at the Lockheed Skunk Works: *Keep It Simple Stupid*. Kelly was also famous for "Be quick, be quiet, be on time," also relevant in our battlefield scenario.

Know Your Enemy

Do you know who your enemy is? Is lung cancer or breast cancer your enemy? Is a parasite in the colon your enemy? Do you think the tumor is the enemy? Have you ever thought that the medical insurance companies or pharmaceutical companies who control healthcare finance and manipulate government regulatory agencies might be an unsuspected enemy?

During the Civil War, Abraham Lincoln said, "I have two great enemies, the Southern army in front of me and the financial institutions in the rear. Of the two, the one in the rear is the greatest enemy."

Who is controlling your medical care? Is it possible that financial control of medical care creates a conflict of interest? Do you want to be at the mercy of the insurance companies and pharmaceutical conglomerates that make decisions about eligibility for cancer care treatments? You can decide on your own. You have a lot more control than you may think.

Know Yourself

What is your overall condition? Are you physically and emotionally fit to fight the battle? What happened to your immune (defense) system that was supposed to act as a surveillance system while the cancer was growing? What kind of environmental toxins have you been exposed to during your lifetime?

Check your biological terrain and fortify any weaknesses in your immune system. Are there any unresolved emotional conflicts slowly eating you alive? You don't need an in-depth psychoanalysis, but be honest with yourself and address any unresolved emotional conflicts. Many people who suffer from unresolved emotional conflict have already given up on life at a subconscious level.

Know Your Terrain

In the military, we want to know the terrain of the battlefields by controlling the entire land, sea, sky, space, night operation and cyberwarfare through command, control and communication. In our battalion, we want to know our biological terrain by measuring the blood, saliva and urine for acid/base (pH), reduction/oxidation potential (rH2) and resistivity (R) and map out the biocybernetic matrix system known to mankind as acupuncture meridians.

We have international law that establishes limits on acceptable wartime conduct. For example, the Geneva Convention and the rules of engagement dictate that we cannot fire first unless we have been attacked. At the same time, we use drones and other means to attack first – acting in violation of the provisions of the laws of war. Does medicine misuse "preemptive strikes" with chemotherapy and radiation aimed at tumors, rather than first detecting and engaging the real sources of conflict and disease?

Medical/Legal/Economic Considerations

Much of integrative medical care is not recognized by insurance companies as legitimate, science-based medicine approved by a panel of experts. Typically, insurance coverage for integrative care is denied, forcing patients to pay for treatment out of their own pockets. Integrative therapies should be cost effective compared to surgery and lifelong medication, and should be available to all.

Sabotage/Counter-Intelligence

Too many patients sabotage themselves with excuses that are equivalent to counter-intelligence. For example, they refuse to get dental work done. Many see dental work as too expensive, yet they pay for a new car or a vacation. Some patients say they will do anything except a gallbladder/liver flush, a colonic or a coffee enema. Other patients may say their oncologist told them they cannot take any vitamins or minerals because they may interfere with their therapies.

Collateral Damage by Friendly Fire

Unintended side effects by friendly fire are a part of war and they are called fratricide. Here's the definition of friendly fire:

"The employment of friendly weapons with the intent to kill the enemy or destroy his equipment or facilities, which results in the unforeseen or unintentional death, injury or damage to friendly personnel."

U.S. Army, Field Manual 17-15, Appendix F

Friendly fire accounts for 25 percent of the body counts in modern warfare. Unfortunately, friendly fire also takes a major toll in cancer care, raising the body count.

An article in *Journal of the American Medical Association (JAMA 2000)* reported there were 225,000 deaths per year from iatrogenic causes – deaths inadvertently caused by a physician, medicine or medical treatment – constituting the third leading cause of death in the United States, after deaths from heart disease and cancer.[6]

Five years later, a 2005 study in the *Journal of Orthomolecular Medicine* found that there were 784,000 deaths caused by iatrogenic medical care at a cost of $280 billion dollars, reporting it as the leading cause of death in the United States.[7]

Public Opinion/Civil Affair/A Family Divided

Win the crowd and win public opinion. Unless you conduct a war with public support, you will have anti-war demonstrations in the street. Opinion also counts in patient families.

As an example, an elderly man with liver cancer, who did not respond to chemotherapy, came to see me. He had six children and they were equally divided over their father's medical care. Three children strongly opposed integrative therapy despite failed standard medical care, and three children were strong supporters of integrative medicine. One of the children was an FBI agent investigating medical fraud who accused me of taking advantage of his father. He was the most vocal and threatened to stop the treatment. I told his father that I would treat him free of charge, so his son could not possibly accuse me of taking advantage.

Due to family pressure, this patient decided not to pursue my medical care, not because he was not interested in my treatment, but because he did not want his children fighting over him at the dinner table. He passed away shortly thereafter. I don't know if I could have helped him. I never had a chance to try integrative therapies because his family disagreed about his choice of therapies.

Cyber Warfare/Military Intelligence

Comedian George Carlin popularized the oxymoron "military intelligence" in the 1970s and 1980s. Today, the U.S. Army Cyber Command (established in October 2010) has the latest electronic/computer software technology to break an enemy's communication system.

Even with the most advanced medical technologies, Western medicine has not embraced the concept of mapping invisible intelligence in the body based on Acupuncture Meridian Assessment. Such an assessment is comparable to breaking an enemy's code using a biomatrix system that is several thousand years old.

Overdiagnosis and Misdiagnosis of Cancer

The National Cancer Institute (NCI) reports that a significant number of people who have undergone treatment for cancer over the past several decades may not have ever actually had the disease. The NCI study identifies overdiagnosis and misdiagnosis of cancer as two major causes of a growing epidemic that has led to unnecessary treatment of otherwise healthy individuals with chemotherapy, radiation and/or surgery.

As an example, breast cancer ductal carcinoma in situ (DCIS) is considered a benign condition. Although DCIS is classified as a stage 0 cancer not indicated for aggressive chemotherapy, I have met many women whose doctors talk or scare them into undergoing chemotherapy.

I've also met men whose doctors told them they have high grade prostatic intraepithelial neoplasia (HGPIN), a type of premalignant precursor to prostate cancer that is not an actual cancer. These same patients were treated as though they had the disease.

By themselves, intelligence and information are not useful. What's critical is what you do with the information. Who controls and monitors decisions for administering chemotherapy and radiation therapy? Once a patient has been told they have cancer, most cannot think clearly. At that point, it is extremely difficult to convince a patient that they are still in control with the power to make their own decisions. Often, they jump into chemotherapy and radiation therapy due to pressure from their doctor.

PSYOPs or Psychological Operations

Psychological Operations or PSYOPs are planned operations to influence an audience's emotions, motives, objective reasoning, and ultimately their behavior.

The National Cancer Institute's position is that cancer is a complex genetic disease. If you have cancer, you will hear this many times, and you'll be told that your primary care physician cannot help you. For the last 40 years, cancer patients have been presented with very limited options:

- Surgery
- Chemotherapy
- Radiation

Based on recent pharmaceutical research, immunotherapy is now being added to the agenda. Unfortunately, it is hard to control its impacts and how the body will respond, attacking the cancer without attacking healthy cells. Success rates are limited, and side effects, including death, are substantial. Doctors and the public are now waking up to this campaign and misinformation about cancer.

Special Operations and Black Ops

War zones always seem to have special operations that are considered top secret black ops. Special operations and black ops are considered to be a violation of the laws of war, yet they exist and we learn about them years later.

It is not uncommon for patients to try all kinds of experimental therapies considered to be "secret formulas" offered by practitioners who practice underground medicine without a proper license. Be aware, and beware.

Post War, Exit Strategy and Prevention of Future War

Preparing an exit strategy is a key part of war planning. Shrinking a tumor with chemotherapy or radiation on the battlefield is not the same as winning the war. We may have won a battle, but we are losing the War on Cancer because we do not have a battle plan.

The medical equivalent of collateral damage and fratricide weakens the immune system while the enemy moves and strikes even stronger in a different location of the body, via "metastasis" or spread of cancer cells. Once you have shrunk cancer, you need to continue therapy to prevent the cancer from coming back. This can be accomplished by altering the biological terrain.

Prevention of war becomes your lifelong commitment. Perpetual war is highly profitable for special interest groups, but the prevention of the next war requires a lifetime commitment to addressing asymmetric threats, changes in lifestyle, a diet based on whole foods, and detoxification.

Force Management

Recognize the area of target is a tumor, but the area of an operation is the whole body with a battle space that includes your family, job, HMO/medical insurance, home environment, religious background and friends that provide support (or lack thereof). The survival rate is based on whether the cancer is early stage or final stage after multiple surgeries, chemotherapy and radiation therapy. The more chemotherapy and radiation your body receives, the less you will be able to respond to nutrition therapy or other treatments.

Early Signs and Symptoms of Cancer

What are the early signs and symptoms of cancer? Most of the early signs are subtle, insidious and often overlooked for many years as a nuisance or inconvenience. Here are common early signs and symptoms of cancer:

- Indigestion
- Sore that does not heal within few weeks
- Change in bowel or bladder habits
- Persistent hoarseness or a cough
- Difficulty swallowing
- Changing size/color or discharge of a skin lesion
- Lump that does not go away

Indigestion is an example of a symptom patients consider to be inconvenient, and many look for a quick treatment such as an anti-acid medication. If you have prolonged indigestion that you're solving with antacid medications, you are blocking the acid production in the stomach that is critical for the breakdown of food into protein, fat and carbohydrates. Our own digestive enzymes also kill bacteria and parasites. Television commercials are saturated with antacid commercials with sleek, misleading information that perpetuates the problem. Instead of an antacid medication, apple cider vinegar mixed with water and sipped during a meal is a natural remedy that works. Some patients take digestive enzymes to help indigestion and acid reflux symptoms.

A New Environment Brings New Health Threats

In ancient societies, people died from accidents, starvation, predation and infectious diseases. In modern industrialized countries, people die from heart disease and cancer, other chronic diseases associated with lifestyle including diabetes and obesity, new infectious diseases, chemicals and neurotoxins, and from complications of medical treatments. Cancer was a rare disease over 200 years ago and an uncommon one 100 years ago.

There has been a rapid change in our environment with industrialization and a shift from acute medical problems to chronic diseases like cancer, heart disease, autoimmune diseases and neurologic disorders that cannot be explained by genetic adaptation or mutations. What are the connections between our new environment and the emerging killers?

Even if we are awake and paying attention to the connection between pollution and chronic diseases, are we overlooking important aspects that might be a trigger? Could there be something that has not been addressed that is right under our noses that could potentially blindside us?

Below are the issues I have found are crucial to turning the tide in the War on Cancer, through detecting and developing a battle plan with each patient. The issues represent problems that need to be addressed as soon as possible at the early stages of disease. I have covered these topics in my first book, and now address them using the expression "asymmetric threats:"

- Parasites and fungi
- Dental problems
- Detoxification
- Heavy metals
- Diet and Nutrition

It is also important to encourage the patient to work on any toxic emotions they may be experiencing, as they will block the journey and quest for health, and be a drag on the immune system.

The word parasite has a different definition and meaning to different people. I am not talking about large human-sized parasites (Para-sapiens) who live, breathe and make profits in Washington, D.C. or too-big-to-fail corporations. I am talking about a parasite as an animal living at the expense of the host, and robbing the host's food. Examples include tapeworms, flukes, Ascaris, Strongyloides, amoeba, protozoa and many unidentified parasites living in the human body as uninvited guests. Parasites are macroorganisms that can also bring additional uninvited guests, such as bacteria, fungi and viruses. When you take care of parasites, the other problems they bring often resolve.

Tumors May Disappear When Meridians Are Balanced

I have observed many patient tumors *spontaneously* disappear while balancing the patient's meridians with:

- Parasite and fungal eradication
- Correction of hidden dental problems
- Heavy metal detoxification
- Elimination of food allergies
- Nutritional support

From the perspective of modern medicine, asymmetric threats come from overlooking hidden dental problems and unrecognized infections, especially parasites and fungi, and from medical treatment itself. Others include environmental toxicities, heavy metals, food allergies, genetically modified foods, and nutritionally depleted junk foods.

Military historians understand that innovative asymmetric tactics have changed the outcomes of battles, as well as world history. To detect and fight invisible parasites, you must adopt asymmetric warfare. Are medical schools and medical scientists training future medical doctors to handle asymmetric biological threats like parasites, heavy metals, environmental pollutions, nutritional deficiencies, and hidden dental problems? I doubt it. Traditional medical use of antibiotics, chemotherapy and radiation therapy are not adequate for asymmetric biological warfare. Immunotherapy and genetic targeting are not enough when they ignore basic principles of a healthy biological terrain and building strength to counter asymmetric threats.

Reassessing Enemies and Friends

It is my conviction that hidden truths will eventually be revealed, just as all hidden toxins will have an impact on the body, brain and health. Einstein once said, "We cannot solve problems by using the same kind of thinking we used when we created them." We must think differently! Learn about and understand the concepts of biological terrain, biocybernetic matrix, Acupuncture Meridian Assessment, and asymmetric warfare.

If we are engaged in the War on Cancer, there are three tasks we need to accomplish:

1. Define the enemy.

2. Use friendly therapies that support the immune system.
3. Understand the battlefield, the biological terrain.

The enemy is not what you think or what you have been told.

My Command Philosophy

I believe command philosophy is unique to every commander based on his or her life experience, personal belief system, and background of military experience. I started as a lieutenant in the U.S. Army Reserve nearly 30 years ago while in medical school, and I witnessed many changes in the medical field and the military.

As part of my training at the Command and General Staff College, we were required to write our own command philosophy. My command philosophy can be summarized as, "Do the right thing the first time. Be willing to adapt to change and do the right thing again." I have seen many medical doctors who did the right thing, but were unable to adapt to new information and new changes in the economic and political environment. When you are no longer able to adapt to change, you cannot "do the right thing."

What I learned nearly 30 years ago in medical school is no longer currently valid, and what I practiced 10 years ago is considered obsolete. What I am practicing now could be considered obsolete and unsound medical practice 10 years in the future. Command philosophy must reflect effective leadership through adaptation to changes in new environments. In addition, while much has changed, it is important to recognize that the cornerstones of our foundation will never change.

Important Values

Command philosophy must also reflect the most important values to an organization: duty, honor, courage, integrity, loyalty, respect, and selfless service. The most important ingredient to carry out these important seven values is leadership. Leadership is fostered through a strong vision of command philosophy.

The History of the Army is a History of Change

When the Berlin Wall came down in 1989, the world changed dramatically, and the impact of that change for the U.S. Army was more than anybody could predict. Since 1991, the U.S. has maintained a Cold-War-level superpower military even though the Cold War has ended. The U.S. military has been engaged in conflict almost continuously. Examples include the Gulf War, regional conflicts in Bosnia, Kosovo and Haiti, followed by a war on terrorism in Afghanistan.

We should not be afraid of change. The history of the Army is a history of change. We have over 220 years of tradition in which the Army has continually changed to meet the needs of the country. Leadership is the key to our strength. We have the most experienced and best-qualified leaders in military history. Moreover, if we understand the challenge of changes in this turbulent new world order, and we are pulling together, there is no limit to what we can accomplish.

Conclusion

It is time to apply these same principles to cancer, chronic illness and medicine. Develop a battle plan to counter asymmetric threats, and rebuild and strengthen your biological terrain so it is friendly to allies instead of harboring hostile enemies that destroy your health. Accept and prepare for the asymmetric paradox. Commit to your journey and quest for health.

Article: Disappearance of the Universe As We Know It for WIMPS - What if Patient Doesn't Really Have Cancer?

This article speaks to the "unknown unknowns" in the universe, and in health and disease. Physicians must develop and patients must execute effective battle plans on their journeys, utilizing the best strategies and tools available.

In case you are not familiar with the history of our universe, NASA's 203 Wilkinson Microwave Anisotropy Probe (WMAP) Spacecraft expedition revealed vital information about our universe. The age of the universe is estimated at 13.7 billion years. The universe is made-up of 4 percent matter consisting of stars, planets and gases, 23 percent exotic "dark matter" detectable by its gravity, and 73 percent "dark energy" detectable by an antigravity force. The size of the universe is unknown; it is expanding and really big. The shape of the universe is perfectly flat – like a pizza.

Roger Penrose, of Oxford University, in the December 2010 issue of *The Economist*, writing about science and technology, states that the Big Bang in which the visible universe began was not actually the beginning of everything that we know of as our universe. It was merely the latest example of a series of such bangs that renew reality when it is getting tired out. More importantly, he thinks that the pre-Big Bang past has left an imprint on the present that can be detected and analyzed.

The imprint in question is in the cosmic microwave background (CMB). CMB is the radiation that fills the whole universe. CMB carries information about what the early universe was like. The CMB is almost but not quite uniform, and known irregularities in it are the seeds from the galaxies from which stars and planets grew.

If Dr. Penrose is correct, there was no Big Bang and much of what people thought they knew about the universe is false. With the best scientific instruments of detection, we can only measure 4 percent of the universe, while 96 percent of the universe is considered to be made of "dark matter and dark energy," which means we don't know what it is, but it is out there.

Five thousand feet below the Black Hills of South Dakota, at the closed-down gold mine town called Lead, a team of scientists and former miners are racing to solve one of the biggest mysteries of physics, dark matter, by using the Large Underground Xenon (LUX) dark matter detector. Most physicists agree that dark matter exists and is made of WIMPs.

WIMP stands for "weakly interacting massive particle." "Massive" does not mean large, but that they have mass and therefore both respond to and cause gravitational pull. "Weakly interacting" means that the particles, despite having mass, nonetheless only rarely interact with matter. WIMPs are electromagnetically neutral which is why we can't see them.

When astronomers find evidence of dark matter, it appears in the universe unevenly distributed. Gravitationally, it behaves like regular matter, and it clumps together in a spherical cloud encompassing most galaxies (*Popular Science*, January 2011).

Why am I bringing up controversial topics in physics? The Big Bang theory in physics is just a theory with a belief system. Maybe it will change to a "Little Bang" theory with many string theories attached to it. With the best medical scientific instruments, we can only measure a small fraction of the human being in the form of blood chemistry, x-ray, CT scan, MRI, or PET scan.

How and why do some of my fibromyalgia patients respond after correcting their dental cavitations (jawbone infections)? Why do some irritable bowel syndrome (IBS) patients respond to antiparasitic medications? Why do chronic fatigue patients respond to combinations of dental work, parasite eradications, and nutritional therapy?

Some of my patients with advanced metastatic cancer documented by tissue biopsy, x-ray and PET scan, with massive tumors, respond to intensive detoxification, nutritional therapies, dental work, and parasite medications. Disappearance of the tumor occurs without targeting to destroy the cancer cells. Is this what we call spontaneous healing or an accidental cure? My book, *Accidental Cure,* addresses these phenomena by explaining the acupuncture meridians and biocybernetics.

What are we missing? New medicine based on a new understanding of biology is here to challenge the basis of Western medicine, which has been dominated by a Newtonian mechanistic view of causes and effects. What happens to the 96 percent of the universe as dark matter and dark energy that we cannot measure with our best scientific instruments? Are they really WIMPs?

What if the cancer patient with a massive tumor did not have cancer? Maybe 96 percent of the tumor mass is not cancer cells, but something else like WIMPs, dark matter, and dark energy? Modern medicine is unlikely to see the importance of treating the whole body in the War against Cancer. Today's cancer establishment rigorously adheres to therapies that have been used for almost 100 years. To most oncologists, the idea is most likely as far-fetched as a disappearance of the universe as we know it.

Part 2
Acupuncture Meridian Assessment: Key Concepts

Chapter 3 Accidental Cure and Acupuncture Meridian Assessment

The human body is a delicate energy system that might be considered analogous to a fine musical instrument such as a violin. The body, it may be said, is part of the symphony of life.

Have you ever wondered why some people who eat organic whole foods, exercise, have a positive mental attitude, and take nutritional supplements suffer from heart attacks and chronic, lingering diseases? How about people who are diagnosed with cancer who you thought were in good health?

Doctors may run a battery of lab tests and come to the conclusion that a patient is physically fit, yet the patient may suffer from unexplainable debilitating fatigue, irritability, mood swings, or migrating pain.

If you're out of tune and out of balance but have perfect lab tests, there may be a missing link in your medical evaluation. Medical doctors may relieve symptoms with medications, but they seldom offer solutions to correct the underlying problems.

When a doctor is in doubt, he/she often blames genetics or calls the symptoms "idiopathic," meaning they don't know what is wrong. In desperation, a physician may even say a patient is malingering – meaning he/she is faking an illness to avoid work. At times, a doctor may also say an illness is "all in his/her head."

Treating the Symptoms of Disease

I have been practicing Internal Medicine for over 30 years. I also worked for an HMO (Health Maintenance Organization) for almost 10 years before I recognized that I was treating the symptoms of disease with medications. The medications I prescribed have similar names that all begin with "anti" including antihypertensive, antianginal, anti-inflammatory, anti-hypercholesterolemia or anti-aging hormone replacements.

The medications never correct the underlying problems, and each medication creates its own side effects that require other medications. Such treatment creates a drug dependency, and medications become medical intervention for the management of symptoms related to that particular disease. In an HMO, the management of a disease is a lucrative business. It turns out that curing a patient is not financially rewarding for the medical-pharmaceutical industry.

An Opportunity for Accidental Cure Must Be Created

I use the words "accidental healing" (that officially includes placebo effects and spontaneous healing) because such "accidents" are a lot more common than you think. What's important to realize is that an opportunity for an "accidental cure" must be created in order for it to happen. In order to do this, one must first understand the biological "terrain" or condition of the body as a whole.

Our mind/body/spirit is unique and infinitely more complex than modern science can comprehend. When an "incurable" patient gets well by some form of healing other than what traditional medicine has to offer, doctors often attribute it to a placebo effect or spontaneous healing. Sometimes, a medical professional will even go into denial by saying they think they made a wrong diagnosis.

Acupuncture Never "Fit" into the Western Medical Model

New York Times reporter James Reston wrote about his experience with acupuncture for pain control when he had an emergency appendectomy during President Nixon's 1972 visit to China. Most physicians dismissed it as a "placebo" effect. Placebos have been accepted by Western medicine since the beginning of the 20th century. They are sugar pills or saline injections that are given to patients in place of drugs and result in therapeutic improvement. Improvement is thought to be due to a patient's faith in the doctor.

Because Western doctors expect to see as many as 30% of patients have therapeutic improvement with a "pharmacologically inert substance," they were quick to assume that acupuncture's benefits were due to placebo. The placebo effect does not explain acupuncture's success on animals, but this point is rarely discussed in the West.

Medicine Among Ancient Societies

Every advanced society has had traditional medical care since the time of antiquity. The civilizations of Egypt, Greece, India, and China each had their own unique medical problems and distinct traditional practices. Today these ancient practices are referred to as Egyptian Antiquity Medicine, Greek Medicine, Ayurvedic Medicine, and Traditional Chinese Medicine.

Hippocrates is best known in Western medicine for his Hippocratic Corpus, Hippocratic Oath, and famous quote from *Of the Epidemics*: "***do no harm.***"[8] Hippocratic physicians practiced medicine with limited medical knowledge. To them, healing was patient-oriented with a focus on rebalancing the "dis-ease" of the patient, rather than overcoming the disease. For example, faced with a fever, one of the most dreaded medical conditions of the time, Hippocratic physicians did not attempt any heroic treatment. They gave general support with boiled barley water, honey, vinegar and bedside attention.

Hippocratic physicians believed in the healing power of nature ("vis medicatrix naturae" in Latin). Drug therapy was considered unpredictable, and those physicians preferred dietary regulation. A most quotable quote from the Hippocratic philosophy reads:

> *"Let your food be your medicine,*
> *Let your medicine be your food."*

Acupuncture Meridian Assessment

Our bodies operate in several different energy realms including bioelectrical and magnetic systems, as well as the familiar biomechanical and biochemical systems.

Einstein's theory of relativity and the quantum theory of uncertainty opened up a new dimension of wave-particle theory, the duality of energy and matter, and the nature and behavior of matter and energy on the atomic and subatomic levels. Humans and all living and non-living things are both matter and energy.

In truth, energy animates life. You might be surprised to learn that pathways of electrical impulses – meridians – run throughout your body, each with a specific frequency. These meridians connect specific organs, sensory organs, joints, teeth and tissues with points located next to the skin, called acupuncture points. Each meridian has an energy frequency that indicates healthy functioning, like a violin string when it is in tune. When the frequency is thrown off, it goes out of tune and does not work as well, indicating disease and dysfunction.

Although electrical and magnetic energies are used in diagnostic tools such as EKG (electrocardiogram) and MRI (magnetic resonance imaging), these tools operate using a "mechanistic" Newtonian view of the body.

In addition to using the standard diagnostic tools, there are other ways of measuring the "energy systems" of the body. I measure the energy in the body's acupuncture meridians – the subtle human energies – in all my patients during their first visit. Acupuncture has been practiced for several thousand years in China and throughout Asia. Currently, the best science cannot explain the origin of the energy in the body's acupuncture meridians. Acupuncture Meridian Assessment, although not considered a diagnostic test, can reveal unique biofeedback information about a patient's energy patterns based on ancient knowledge of acupuncture and meridian flows of the body, updated to the biocybernetic and digital worlds.

In my practice, I explain to new patients that I compare a human body that is sick to a violin that is out of tune. This makes a doctor the person who does the tuning. The medical name I give to the job of tuning is called Acupuncture Meridian Assessment (AMA). A violin metaphor helps explain the concept of energy medicine that is not widely understood in the United States. When all the strings are in tune, the violin is working to play the best sounds it was crafted to produce. If any of the strings are out of balance, it is no longer working in harmony and is out of tune. This concept was explained in depth in my first book.

In the body, when all of the meridians are balanced, the body's interconnected systems are working well, producing harmony and health. Problems along the meridians, which connect specific organs, joints, tissues, teeth and more, will show up in high or low readings, and indicate infection, inflammation, degeneration, and underlying causes of diseases.

When used by an experienced practitioner, the instrument used for Acupuncture Meridian Assessment detects electrical field disturbance signals that can indicate hidden dental problems, environmental toxicities, hidden parasite infections, and other "imbalances" of the body. These "imbalances" are indications that the biocybernetic system is compromised and not functioning at its optimum capacity.

The human body is a delicate energy system that might be considered analogous to a fine musical instrument such as a violin. The body, it may be said, is part of the symphony of life.

Recommendations That May Seem Odd

My assessment and recommendations may seem odd for some patients, and may provoke doubt and skepticism. For example, based on Acupuncture Meridian Assessment, a physical exam, laboratory tests, and a medical history, extraction of an asymptomatic root canal might be recommended and a patient's arthritis or chest pain may improve. For another patient, a treatment for parasites may improve not only their abdominal pain or irritable bowel, but may also relieve knee pain, sciatic pain, or headache. For some people diagnosed with multiple sclerosis (MS), a treatment for parasites may even dissolve brain lesions.

Another patient may receive EDTA chelation therapy for heavy metal toxicity, and their chest pain may go away. For yet another patient, when one or a combination of the above seemingly unrelated therapies are carried out, cancer may go into "spontaneous" remission. These phenomena are very difficult to explain by deductive, Newtonian-based western medical science.

Our body/mind/spirit operates as a whole system, not simply a collection of parts. It operates in a closed biomechanical, chemical, and electrical system within an open biocybernetic energy field.

The Dilemma of Evidence-Based Medicine

Modern medicine has evolved through the paradigm of the random clinical trial. A subgroup of patients with a similar disease diagnosis – collection of symptoms based on medical history, observation and lab tests – are given a drug, and a comparable random control group is given a placebo. When the drug, device or procedure being tested shows safety and a level of effectiveness in alleviating the symptoms on average across the group of patients in the trial – compared to the control group – it is approved for use. Once approved, it may be incorporated into guidelines of the relevant specialty group, and for payment by insurance companies and pharmacy benefit managers.

In contrast, energy medicine detects medical problems and helps guide treatment approaches not by common symptoms and disease diagnosis, but by underlying causes. Therefore, one patient's MS symptoms may respond to chelation of heavy metals and removal of an infected root canal, while another patient's MS may respond to antiparasitic medications. Therefore, standard medical trials will not capture these results.

Conventional medicine would say energy medicine is not evidence-based medicine. Instead, it would be more accurate to say that energy medicine is based on the evidence of the patient's response – individualized, personalized medicine – not the patient disease group's response.

Assessing the Whole System

On your first visit, I may not focus on your list of complaints or symptoms. You may think I am ignoring your complaints, but I am working to create a "pattern" of the body's energy system based on Acupuncture Meridian Assessment. Rather than looking at your "collection of symptoms," I look at your entire system to correct any "disturbed" or "imbalanced" meridians. The body's immune system tries to heal itself as long as input and output are corrected.

Discovering and correcting the underlying problems allows your body to heal itself regardless of your diagnosis. I call this healing phenomenon "accidental cure." Having experienced it first-hand, I know that this process works. The first time a patient witnesses this process they are often surprised, amazed, and delighted. It is only then that they truly understand the phenomenon. If you can identify the underlying causes of your problems and balance the meridians, you may achieve an "accidental cure."

Patients Who Are Candidates for Extreme Medicine

One of my favorite articles is called, "Extreme Medicine for Extreme Patients." Many patients come to see me with a whole list of medical conditions and unusual complaints. They have seen numerous medical doctors and integrative/complementary/holistic practitioners or different specialists. They have medically unexplained symptoms (MUS). Some of these patients come to see me with the claim, "Doctor, I am weird! Nobody knows what is wrong with me."

Doctors have often labeled these patients as difficult, extreme, or weird. Many of these patients are desperate to regain their lives back. They're looking for "whatever it takes" to get well. These patients are good candidates for what I call "extreme medicine for extreme patients" or "extraordinary medicine for extraordinary patients." I don't call them difficult – I call them extraordinary, and we must rise to the challenge with new tools and techniques.

So, what is considered to be "extreme medicine" in today's standard medical care? Is it acupuncture or yoga? Not really. Some women will go through a preventive double mastectomy based on a family history of breast cancer and genetic testing. That is what I call extreme medicine. Heart bypass operations or heart transplants might have been considered extreme medicine 30 years ago, but by today's standards, these operations are considered to be no big deal. Chemotherapy, radiation therapy, and bone marrow transplants for cancer patients are also considered to be standard treatments by today's standards.

Standard Medical Treatment in My Office

Although most physicians ridicule integrative and complementary medical doctors when they prescribe herbs to clean out the bowel, liver, and kidney, most of my patients start with bowel cleansing, kidney and liver cleansing, as well as parasite cleansing. Patients are also evaluated and mapped out for their biocybernetic energy matrix based on an Acupuncture Meridian Assessment. Hair tissue mineral analysis and food allergy tests are also standards, used to design nutritional and dietary recommendations.

When you apply all these unusual modalities and therapies in the right sequence, you'll often observe spontaneous healing or an accidental cure. The body begins to repair and correct itself when you remove underlying toxic conditions.

Having an unexplained medical condition does not mean you're weird. However, you might be a candidate for the extreme medicine that I have described, or extraordinary medicine for extraordinary patients. You don't want to be a casualty of the "AcciDental Blow Up in Medicine." You'll need a physician who is knowledgeable about Accidental Cure and many unusual integrative therapies. Hopefully, he isn't too weird.

Acupuncture Meridian Assessment Does Not Use Needles

It is quite common for new patients to assume that there are needles used in the Acupuncture Meridian Assessment work that I do. My work with the EAV device (used to perform AMA, the name comes from electroacupuncture according to Dr. Voll) measures skin resistivity at 50 of the 500 classical acupuncture points, and there are no needles involved. Organs, joints and teeth are all connected to the acupuncture meridians. Physical symptoms in the body are reflected in the mouth, and biological dentists understand the connection between weak organs and problem teeth. The points that I measure run along the system of channels or major meridians that channel energy to the organs of the body.

Measuring the frequency of the microcurrent at each acupuncture point, a reading of 45-55 is considered balanced on a scale of 0-100. Higher readings indicate the presence of acute infection and inflammation, and lower readings, chronic inflammation and degeneration. Depending on the potential problem suspected, prescription medications (and other remedies) can be added to the test plate. If they rebalance the microcurrent toward the midpoint, that is an indication of the likelihood that they will be an effective treatment. This process can also be used to help determine the dosages and combination of medications.

I hope this chapter excites you and prepares you to explore new concepts: Acupuncture Meridian Assessment, biocybernetics, biological terrain, chelation for heavy metal toxicity, dental-medical connections, parasites, fungi, food allergies, nutritional therapy, detoxification, and more. After you've read the next chapter, you will have the foundation to move forward with a physician using new forensic tools to help develop a strategic, targeted and effective battle plan toward an "accidental cure."

Article: Curing the Incurable by Measuring the Immeasurable: Mapping the Invisible Body by Biocybernetics

This article will help tie it all together, by combining some of the history behind "measuring the immeasurable" with stories of four patients I have seen with different health problems.

Is it possible to map the invisible body? In Germany, there is an emerging biomedical discipline called biocybernetics which has been measuring the invisible, energy field of the human body. Biocybernetics is a key component of the broader field of Energy Medicine in Europe. It is actually not a new idea, but an old concept that has been given a new name. Biocybernetic matrix is a modern term for the acupuncture meridian system and the related field of Acupuncture Meridian Assessment developed by Reinhold Voll, MD in the 1950's in Germany.

In 1895, German physicist Wilhelm C. Roentgen discovered mysterious rays capable of passing through the human body. Because of their unknown nature, he called them x-rays. Because of his discovery, he was awarded the first Nobel Prize in Physics in 1901. X-rays are electromagnetic waves situated between UV (ultraviolet) light and gamma rays on the wavelength scale. Marie Curie built x-ray machines for French doctors in World War I. They helped detect the location of bullets, shrapnel and broken bones in the body which, of course, were invisible to the human eye. X-rays revolutionized medicine and the rest "became history."

Measuring the "immeasurable" human energy field by utilizing the biocybernetic matrix of the body's meridian systems will have a similar impact to discovering x-rays. Every day, I see patients who have been to one doctor after another, one hospital after another, trying to figure out why they are so sick. None of the various specialists these patients have seen seem to have any clue as to what is wrong with them.

Marie, a 19-year-old college student, came to see me with a history of chest and leg pain for over a year. Although she saw several cardiologists, an orthopedic surgeon, and other specialists, none of her doctors gave her a definite diagnosis or treatment plan, even after extensive medical tests and evaluations. When I saw her, her physical exam was normal. I checked 54 acupuncture points as part of my meridian assessment, and her dental area showed pathology. A further detailed evaluation revealed her problem was arising from tooth #17 – an old wisdom tooth socket.

Marie's problem was a dental-related medical problem, which is an all-too-common, often overlooked situation. Medical doctors cannot understand or fix her problem. She needs an oral surgeon to correct the problem. I could not guarantee that oral surgery would fix her chest and leg pain. However, based on over 25 years of practicing Acupuncture Meridian Assessment, I told her I was 85-90% confident that her symptoms would resolve when the dental problem was properly fixed.

This is not an isolated event. I've had multiple cases of unexplainable chest pain that respond favorably to cleaning out an old infected wisdom tooth area. The power of biocybernetics and meridian assessments is used to reveal the true cause of underlying illnesses. Once the true cause was revealed, a specific treatment plan can be implemented and, sometimes almost unbelievably, healing is achieved.

Joanne, an elderly woman with fibromyalgia is another example. An evaluation revealed that her diagnosis of fibromyalgia wasn't really fibromyalgia. Her evaluation indicated that she should be treated with parasite medications. She fully responded and her unexplainable pain disappeared.

Jill's asthma disappeared after an extraction of a root canal. Susan's asthma was eliminated with parasite medications. These two different women with the same condition (asthma) required two distinct approaches because the individual condition of each person was unique.

Mary, a young woman with acute panic attacks and a nervous breakdown responded to the removal of her "silver" colored dental fillings and recovered her mental health. Note: "silver" dental amalgam fillings are approximately 50% mercury.

None of these patients responded to traditional medical care because their medical evaluations weren't addressing the true cause of their ill health. Instead, they were simply heavily medicated to control their symptoms. They were considered incurable and advised to learn to live with their illness because doctors could not determine what was wrong with them.

Quite a few patients come from all over the United States. This includes a sizable group from Iowa who drive 7-8 hours to see me. They do so because they realize they are not getting better, even after going to the Mayo Clinic. After extensive visits to this Midwestern institution, they need a different outlook on their health and healing. I am always grateful to the Mayo Clinic for their extensive medical evaluations. They have one of the best medical systems available based on Western medical science, and they utilize every known test at their disposal.

After these individuals have been evaluated by the Mayo Clinic without a clear diagnosis, I have the opportunity to evaluate them from an "outside the box" viewpoint. I have repeatedly noticed an emerging pattern of overlooked causes in modern medical diagnoses. The most common neglected areas are: hidden dental-related medical problems, heavy metal toxicity, nutritional deficiencies, parasite problems, and a general lack of understanding of the importance of detoxification of the colon, liver and kidney.

How do I know these problems are the missing links? By understanding biocybernetics and measuring the acupuncture meridian systems in the body's invisible energy matrix. The human body is like a fine-tuned musical instrument that requires constant tuning and calibration to keep one in optimal health.

We desperately need "connections for optimal health" or links that integrate Western-based medical science and the emerging knowledge of biocybernetics through Acupuncture Meridian Assessment. X-rays eventually became less mysterious and later contributed to major advancements in medicine. By combining these disciplines, we can truly "cure the incurable" by "measuring the immeasurable" human energy fields. Just as violins need to be tuned before they are played, the body needs similar tuning.

Chapter 4 Biological Terrain and Biocybernetic Medicine

The body's ability to heal is dependent on its internal environment.

This chapter brings together two concepts that are cornerstones of my practice. Because of medical politics, the concept of biological terrain is foreign to conventionally-trained medical doctors, and biocybernetic medicine is a cutting-edge concept that has become popular with integrative medical doctors in Europe. Both concepts are little known among conventionally trained physicians in the United States.

The Health of the Body's Internal Environment

The concept of biological terrain has been around for many years. It originated with a contemporary of Louis Pasteur's named Claude Bernard (1813-1878) who developed the idea that the body's ability to heal is dependent on its internal environment. Although Bernard developed the original concept of the biological terrain, a medical doctor named Antoine Béchamp (1816-1908) is largely responsible for a more complete theory of biological terrain.

Béchamp built on Barnard's idea and said that health and disease revolve around a concept called "pleomorphism." While Pasteur was promoting the germ theory idea that disease is due to single, fixed-state microbes, Béchamp discovered tiny microorganisms that are "pleomorphic" or "many formed." Pleomorphic microorganisms are found to be present in all things, whether living or dead. In Béchamp's view, these microorganisms are capable of taking on a number of forms, depending on the chemistry of their environment (the body of the host), or the biological terrain.

Modern Medicine Favored Pasteur's Germ Theory

Louis Pasteur is widely known for his germ theory that became the foundation of modern medicine, mostly due to the wide use of antimicrobial remedies. In the second half of the nineteenth century, Pasteur, a French chemist, competed with a German doctor named Robert Koch in an odd "Franco-German" microbial war. The scientists worked diligently to prove that their respective country was superior. In 1885, Pasteur's goal was to solve the problem of human disease, and he developed a successful vaccine for rabies. As a result of this achievement, newspapers funded the Pasteur Institute in Paris that made Pasteur the victor. Indirectly, the rivalry between Pasteur and Koch produced a method for making vaccines and solidified the theory that microbes caused disease.

Understanding Biological Terrain as the Cause of Disease

Today, many scientists understand that Pasteur's germ theory is misguided. In contrast to Pasteur, Bernard and Béchamp believed that disease is a function of biology, and illness is the result of multiple changes that take place in the body when metabolic processes are thrown off. Germs are actually symptoms of a weakened terrain that becomes vulnerable to harmful microorganisms.

Biological terrain may be compared to a garden that requires an understanding of soil conditions. Gardeners who grow healthy fruits and vegetables understand that a plant's environment will determine whether the plant is healthy. They know a garden is much more than a plot of land where seeds are planted. A healthy crop requires an in-depth knowledge of the seeds, nutrients, fertilizers, water drainage, and sunlight. It also requires an understanding of how insects, weeds, molds, and fungi affect the soil and plants.

Managing a healthy biological terrain in the human body is similar to raising healthy vegetables. If the body is fed a diet that provides adequate amounts of vitamins and minerals, if it is nurtured with love and given an adequate amount of exercise, rest, and sleep, the body, like a healthy garden, can flourish with vitality and support a strong immune system. When your immune system is strong and your biological terrain is balanced, you can ward off infections and stay healthy.

Pasteur's germ theory is the foundation of modern medicine's triumph over infectious diseases, but it is also the cause of antibiotic resistance and the development of new and emerging super bugs. The germ theory states that germs are airborne, and specific germs cause specific diseases. This theory led to treatment plans that are designed to eliminate what is believed to be the underlying problem – the disease-causing germs.

Stressors That Can Disturb Your Biological Terrain

As reported in *Accidental Cure*, the most common stressors that can disturb your biological terrain are:

- Hidden Dental Problems
- Heavy Metal Toxicity and Environmental Chemicals
- Parasites, Fungi, and New Emerging Infections
- Allergies
- Poor Diet and Nutrition
- Genetically Modified Organisms (GMOs)

- Lack of Adequate High Quality Water
- Psychological Stress and Negative Emotions
- Medical Therapy and Medications
- Vaccinations
- Structural Imbalance
- Inactivity
- Scars
- Lack of Natural Sunlight and Cosmic Rays
- Electromagnetic Pollution

Biophoton Theory

A biophoton is a photon of light that is emitted from a biological system that can be detected with biological probes. Professor Fritz-Albert Popp, PhD, a theoretical physicist and biophysicist from Germany, is considered the father of biophoton theory.

Popp's work on biophotons goes back to Russia in the 1920s when Russian embryologist Alexander Gurwitsch reported "ultra-weak" photon emissions from living tissues in the ultraviolet range of the spectrum. Fritz Popp and a young graduate student name Bernard Ruth took Gurwitsch's work much further when they built a high-sensitivity emission photometer that was capable of mapping the light or biophotons given off by living systems. They counted biophotons given off by test substances and discovered:

- Vegetables contaminated with heavy metals showed a decreased photon count.
- Tomatoes stored at cold temperatures showed decreased biophoton emissions that decreased even further with longer storage times.
- Photons given off by eggs from captive chickens were lower than from eggs obtained from free-range chickens.

Popp also measured biophotons given off from the human body and saw high photon emissions coming from the hands of an internationally acclaimed healer named Rosalyn Bruyere when she focused her healing energy, compared to light given off when she was resting. Popp suspected that the source of these biophotons was DNA and theorized that each organ and each cell has its own specific spectra, as well as specific disease-producing oscillations with characteristic frequencies. Oscillation refers to a cycle associated with the wave phenomena of light.

The preservation of the healthy oscillation is dependent on the resonating capacity of the cell, organ, tissue, or the whole body. When the resonating capacity is disturbed, incoherent, or inappropriate, disease can develop. Popp discovered that disease has its own electromagnetic waves, and traced tumor problems back to a loss of coherence in the biophoton field.

All Living Organisms Possess Complex Electromagnetic Fields

The new breakthroughs in medicine will come from understanding the biophysics and biocybernetics of cells and organs, not only from the Human Genome Project. Here's what scientists know about the biocybernetics of cells and organs:

- All living organisms possess complex electromagnetic fields and an invisible body.
- Biophotons trigger all biochemical reactions in the living cell.
- Electromagnetic fields disappear completely with death.

Dr. Franz Morell, MD from Germany said, "The oscillation (frequency) of the universe is the cause of the phenomenon called LIFE." These oscillations bring both health and disease. Without electromagnetic oscillations, life is probably inconceivable. Oscillations have four dimensions: length, width, height, and time. Self-healing requires an active cancellation of pathological oscillations and a rebalancing of a disturbed equilibrium.

For those interested in more reading in this area, consider Dr. Robert O. Becker, *The Body Electric: Electromagnetism and The Foundation of Life*, Dr. Richard Gerber, *A Practical Guide to Vibrational Medicine*, Dr. Jerry L. Tennant, *Healing is Voltage: The Handbook*, Claude Swanson, *Life Force, The Scientific Basis: Volume 2 of the Synchronized Universe*, James L. Oschman, *Energy Medicine: The Scientific Basis*, and Carolyn McMakin's *The Resonance Effect* (discussed in my article below).

Here are some interesting points that connect the oscillations in biocybernetics with acupuncture meridians:

- An information exchange within a living organism can only be transmitted by oscillations that move at the speed of light (Popp).
- We are living in the matrix of a biocybernetic system.
- The oscillations of the organs are present on the acupuncture points in a bunched and concentrated form.

The frequency spectrum of an organ is conducted via the meridians and can be detected at the acupuncture points. Nearly the whole oscillation spectrum of the body exists in the palms of the hands and the soles of the feet.

Invisible Body Map of the Biocybernetic Matrix

To my amazement, we already have an "invisible body map of the biocybernetic matrix" in the acupuncture meridian system taught in traditional Chinese medicine (TCM) and the chakra system taught in Ayurvedic medicine. Acupuncture Meridian Assessment (AMA), also known as electroacupuncture according to Dr. Voll (EAV), is one of the most effective ways to learn about the biocybernetic system. It provides a physical means to measure invisible energy functions unknown to Western medicine.

When you can understand biological terrain and measure biocybernetic regulation of the body, you can detect hidden dental infections, parasites, allergies, heavy metals and toxins in the body and start a treatment plan that seems almost impossible in the context of current medical science. All of this makes my type of practice seem magical for new patients and highly suspicious for my medical colleagues in academia or clinical practice. For me, the biocybernetic medicine component of my practice is fascinating, fun, and rewarding. Best of all, it never gets boring. It provides an invaluable forensic tool to help identify and counteract the asymmetric threats causing cancers and chronic illnesses.

Article: FSM, AMA and Pain: Spooky Parasites, Fungal and Dental Entanglements

This article gives more background on the energetic dimension in medicine in the context of related disciplines and an example of the application of Frequency Specific Medicine in pain control.

Would you like to get into the world of quantum weirdness and spooky healing? Treating pain is a huge topic these days. We have a growing opioid crisis because conventional medicine often fails at diagnosing and treating pain. What if I told you there were alternatives that can work much better? And that they involve spooky entanglements?

In September, I attended a Master class for Frequency Specific Microcurrent (FSM) practitioners in Portland, Oregon. We had a unique experience of evaluating Connie, a 24-year-old woman with unusual shoulder dystonia, Vagus nerve dysfunction, and muscular spasm from brachial plexus injury after a car accident. Master FSM practitioner Carolyn McMakin, DC did an amazing job of restoring her function and alleviating her pain using variable specific frequencies in a short time. Seeing is believing!

I also had an opportunity to evaluate Connie with Acupuncture Meridian Assessment (AMA), which is derived from German-based biological medicine and Eastern acupuncture. From my assessment, her problems were coming from whiplash-related dental TMJ/bite issues preventing her trigeminal nervous system from firing properly, and from her allergy/immunology system. I did a simple dental bite adjustment using an impromptu sugar packet to correct her bite, and her tight biceps became more relaxed.

FSM therapy was developed by McMakin and Harry Van Gelder, DO, ND. She refined the technique by using specific frequencies for neuromuscular-myofascial pain. To learn more, see Carolyn McMakin's book, *The Resonance Effect: How Frequency Specific Microcurrent Is Changing Medicine*. For information on FSM's historical roots, see Upton Sinclair's essay, "The House of Wonder," and my article on it, "Frequency Specific Microcurrent (FSM) Therapy: The House of Wonder by a Quack."

A chiropractor specializing in FSM, McMakin has successfully treated many difficult cases. Effectiveness of FSM has been documented in academic journals[9] and at major hospitals, including the Cleveland Clinic.[10] Today, FSM is classified as a TENS (transcutaneous electrical nerve stimulation) unit by the U.S. Food and Drug Administration (FDA).[11]

FSM and AMA are two of the leading methods used in Energy Medicine for evaluation and treatment of complex multisystem failure patients, including those with intractable pain. How to explain them? In Energy Medicine, the field of quantum biology is leading theoretical biology to understand quantum mechanics at the submolecular biological level. As Johnjoe McFadden and Jim Al-Khalili write in the *New York Times* bestseller, *Life on the Edge: The Coming Age of Quantum Biology*, plants use chlorophyll as a quantum effect to capture the energy of the sun, photons, for photosynthesis. Migrating birds use quantum effects to sense magnetic fields using built-in magnetoreceptors for their journey. Read more on life itself in Nick Lane, *The Vital Question.*

Einstein's successors have focused their quest for a "theory of everything" on string theory – the idea that the fundamental constituents of matter are tiny stringlike objects vibrating at different frequencies. The more you investigate quantum biology, the more you get used to the idea, and to words like quantum weirdness and quantum entanglement. For example, particles that were once close but are later separated as far as at the opposite sides of the universe are still connected. In effect, prodding one particle would prompt its distant partner to jump instantaneously. Einstein, who gave us the concept of black holes, warped space-time, and gravitational waves, refused to accept it. He derided it as "spooky action at a distance or spooky entanglement."

Physicists now know that quantum particles can have instantaneous long-range links. Metaphysically, it means we, Mankind and others are connected throughout the universe by waves, particles and frequencies. In fact, we are waves, particles and frequencies. Coincidences, serendipity and accidents are not really coincidental or accidental. It is a part of the spooky entanglement called Life.

Learning about and using FSM and teaching AMA evaluation on Connie in a funky hotel in Portland, Oregon was coincidental serendipity or quantum entanglement of spooky action at a distance. She had multiple physical traumas and very unusual physical symptoms, with injuries to both her vagus (autonomic nervous system-ANS) and trigeminal (dental) nerves.

The cranial trigeminal and vagus nerves are two separate nerves controlling different parts of the body, yet related like one universe. They react spontaneously to the other side of the system in a way similar to what Einstein called spooky entanglement. You can read more in my articles, "Leaky Gut, Leaky Brain: Mind/Body Connection for Irritable Bowel and Irritable Mind," and, "Death Certificate for the Unknown Cause: AcciDental Blow Up in Medicine." Surprisingly, dental is connected to the rest of the body, and fungi and parasites may entangle your brain.

Chapter 5 Medical Acupuncture Meridian Assessment in Action

The most common port of entry is the oral cavity.

Acupuncture Meridian Assessment (AMA) gives assistance in detecting and treating medical problems. In my experience, parasites and fungus often present strongly in the initial evaluation, and should be treated in the first round. The four articles below give examples of how major meridian systems are tied into clinical evaluation and treatment.

The 12 meridians from Traditional Chinese Medicine are: Lung, Large Intestine, Stomach, Spleen, Heart, Small Intestine, Bladder, Kidney, Pericardium, Triple Warmer, Gallbladder, and Liver. The Governing Vessel runs along the back median line of the body, and the Conception Vessel along the front median line. I have included classical illustrations of the Gallbladder, Heart and Large Intestine meridians. The fourth case concerns the dental and allergy points, which are not classical meridians, but were discovered later by Dr. Reinhold Voll, and are used in German Biological Medicine.

Gallbladder Meridian: Therapeutic Illusion on Lyme, Chronic Fatigue, IBS and Autism

Without my knowledge, a mother shared her antiparasitic medications with her son, and he began to emerge from autism. Although I do not see children, I insisted he follow up; he is now fully recovered. A military case of IBS is also described. Gallbladder and intestinal problems are often linked to parasites.

Many times, my patients surprise me. I learn things from them in unexpected ways. An unusual example is a mother-son case of chronic fatigue and autism. Nancy, a 39-year-old registered nurse from Texas, came to see me for weird neurological symptoms with numbness of body, coughing, brain fog, exhaustion, and IBS-like symptoms. My Acupuncture Meridian Assessment indicated 15 out of 40 meridians were out of balance.

Major disturbances came from her **large intestine, small intestine, allergy, and lymphatic meridians**. I started Nancy on the parasite medications ivermectin, pyrantel pamoate, and praziquantel. She noticed a dramatic improvement in her condition with increased energy, no burning sensation, and improved cognition.

Without my knowledge, she decided, out of desperation, to give part of her parasite medications to her five-year-old son diagnosed with severe autism. He was non-verbal and had focal seizures.

Nancy reported this action to me, along with her son's response: a dramatic improvement in his behavior. He started "talking" after taking his mom's parasite medications.

I had to reprimand Nancy for treating her son without a proper medical evaluation. However, I was also impressed by her description of the dramatic improvement of her son's autistic behavior. I insisted on evaluating the child (after the parasite medication given by his mom), and his gallbladder and nervous system meridians were still out of balance. I put him on different rounds of parasite and fungal medications, nystatin, fluconazole and nitazoxanide, to rebalance the rest of the meridians. He also had very high mercury exposure which was addressed. This was most likely from his mom, who also had a high mercury level.

I then saw both of them again. The child's Autism Treatment Evaluation Checklist (ATEC) score dropped from 109 (severe autism) to 6 (considered normal), according to his mom. The ATEC was developed in 1999, not as a diagnostic evaluation but as a way for researchers to evaluate the effectiveness of various treatments for autistic children.

Update

Two years later, Nancy reports: "My son is completely recovered. He's laughing, playing, reading, writing, and has more friends than any child on the block! His intelligence and IQ are astounding but his sense of humor and compassion will blow you away. We are beyond blessed and if it had not been for Dr. Yu, we would not have this child that we have today!!"

I've written several articles on autism, including, "AutismOne on Healing Autism," and "Autism and Autism Spectrum Disorder." I do not treat autism. I treat the underlying problems based on AMA. Most autistic children have disturbances of intestinal and gallbladder meridians.

*   *   *

Ten years ago, at the Combat Support Hospital in Germany, I saw a retired U.S. Army Special Forces warrant officer whom I treated for irritable bowel syndrome. After several previously unsuccessful rounds of meds from other doctors, she positively responded to parasite medications that I prescribed. She even presented me with a special medallion from the 1st Special Forces Group (Airborne). She spread the word to the network of Special Forces for those suffering from IBS to look for parasite problems.

Within the military, IBS is one of many underappreciated burdens. Many soldiers who serve overseas develop "travelers' diarrhea," which is one of the main causes of illness, lost duty days, and compromised missions. A lot of Special Forces are silently suffering from IBS because they are afraid to speak out about their problems for fear of a medical discharge since there is no cure. They may have acquired IBS during their "survival training." It may then have been compounded by overseas operations in many hostile environments and the traumatic stress of combat operations.

*   *   *

The gallbladder meridian is one of the longest and most complex meridians. It partly controls movement, the autonomic nervous system, and cognition. Disturbance of the **gallbladder meridian** has been associated with migraine headache, concentration problems, eye/ear problems, neck pain, indigestion, abdominal pain with nausea, and hip, knee or foot pain.

The gallbladder meridian influences our **central nervous system**: mesencephalon including the center of sleep and waking rhythm, diencephalon sleep center, cranial nerves involving the optic and trigeminal nerves, parasympathetic nervous system including ciliary optic ganglion, vagus nerve in the medulla oblongata, and the cranial part of the sympathetic nervous system. The **gallbladder and liver meridians are paired meridians**. The paired circuitry meridians are the triple warmer (hormonal regulator) and pericardium (circulation) meridians. See Figure 1.

Figure 1. The Gallbladder Meridian

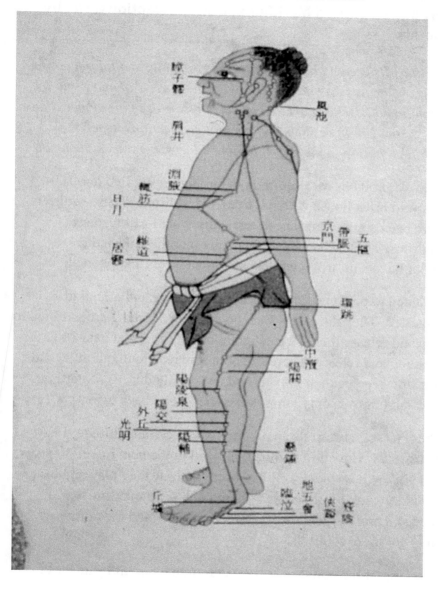

Heart Meridian: Portals of Entry for Squirrels and Dragons – Paired Meridians, Dental Infections, Heavy Metals

Squirrels created havoc in my attic. Same for dental infections, heavy metals and parasites – so many portals of entry into the human body! The heart and small intestine are paired meridians, and can have surprising dental connections which fuel inflammation in the heart, joints, kidneys, nervous system, etc.

I have a problem with squirrels in our home. We live in a 100-year-old brick house with tall trees and squirrels. These squirrels have been a major nuisance, especially what I call teenager squirrels. These teenager squirrels get into the attic and create major havoc, destroying piles of storage boxes and phone lines.

I wanted to poison or shoot them but my wife and grandkid protested. They thought it was too cruel. We hired a professional to trap and release them. We caught nine squirrels and paid $900 for trapping and release. There is a hole somewhere in our attic, and our attic became their playground, especially during wintertime. The solution was only temporary. They came back again.

These teenage squirrels are playful with a certain attitude: smart and sneaky. How do I know? I've lived in the house over 30 years, and got to know them well by observing how they play and move around. I couldn't figure out where the hole in our attic was. I needed a professional roofer or repairman to find the portals of entry for these squirrels.

Speaking of the portal of entry, microorganisms and parasites may penetrate into the human body through skin, eyes, nasal cavities and sinuses, pharynx, bronchi, lungs, oral cavity and the teeth, digestive tract, urinary system, and genitalia. Dental issues and parasites have been my main focus when patients are not responding to standard medical care and not getting well.

The most common portal of entry is the **oral cavity**, that is, any dental-related area. The distance between the **upper dental area to the brain** and the **lower dental area to the thyroid** is about 10 cm, depending on the location of the dental infection. Dental problems such as mercury-containing dental amalgams, root canals, implants, cavitations, and periodontal infections are usually only addressed by dentists. Most medical professionals are not looking at dental issues as hidden medical problems.

A neurologist from Sweden, Patrick Stortebecker, MD, PhD, addressed the principles of the shortest pathway and the portal of entry of infection. In his book, *Dental Caries as a Cause of Nervous Disorders* (1982), he described gold crowns as **Golden Mausoleums**. He also emphatically pointed out that the cranial-dental vertebral vein and pelvic vertebral veins do not have valves, and are a "valveless vein system." They are susceptible to the backflow of venous blood contaminated with infected microorganisms and toxins, providing entry to the brain, brainstem and lower spinal cord. His ideas have never been widely accepted by the medical or dental professions. I bought his book for one cent on Amazon; it is now quite expensive. It is one of the best books I've read on dental-medical-neurological connections.

Dental infections and heavy metals have propensities to settle in and cause **inflammation** in the **heart, gastrointestinal and genitourinary tracts, joints, kidneys, and endocrine/nervous** system. Stefan had an infection in his jawbone area at tooth #17 – an old wisdom tooth area – which corresponds to the heart meridian, and at two root canals at teeth #8 and #20, which correspond to the urogenital/prostate and lymph/spleen meridians. See the Tooth-Organ Meridian Chart in Chapter 6.

My recommendation was to see a biological dentist to remove his two root-canal-treated teeth #8 and #20, and an oral surgeon to operate and clean out the jawbone at wisdom tooth area #17. I also recommended tinidazole, an antiprotozoal parasite medication, for Stefan's bladder/prostate meridian disturbance. Protozoal parasites are very common urogenital infections. Intrauterine devices (IUDs) can also be a focal point for women to develop infections.

A disturbance of the **heart meridian** often comes from silent (painless) **wisdom teeth extraction sites.** These infections are often the overlooked cause of **unexplainable symptoms** of fatigue, headache, arthritic pain, heart problems, insomnia, neurological symptoms, hormonal imbalances, emotional and psychological disturbances, intestinal problems, and facial pain. I wrote a short article on this topic, "Wisdom Teeth, Undetected Tooth Infections and Incurable Medical Symptoms."

The **heart** and **small intestine** meridians are **paired meridians.** Paired circuitry meridians also include the kidney and bladder meridians. If you cannot figure out the portal of entry of squirrels in your house, the damage will magnify. It could grow from a squirrel into a dragon.

I am going to call the roof repair man to fix the portal of entry of squirrels into the attic. If you have incurable medical symptoms, I recommend that you see an MD and biological dentist "team" who understand the Golden Mausoleum of dental-medical connections. See Figure 2.

Figure 2. Heart Meridian

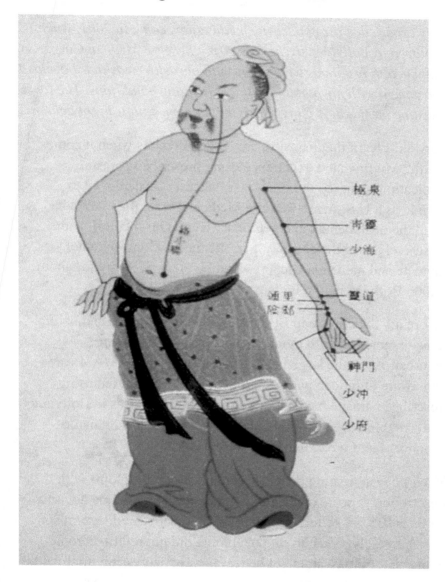

Large Intestine Meridian: U.S. Army Targets Demons

My experience using parasite medications came in 2001, when I deployed to Bolivia with the U.S. Army Reserve Medical Corps. So many health problems went away with parasite meds that I decided to try them with my patients with challenging conditions. The large intestine meridian is paired with the lung meridian; Fight demons!

How did I learn that parasites are hidden demons when it comes to health? My firsthand experience using prescribed parasite medications came in the year 2001, when I was deployed to Bolivia as a U.S. Army Reserve Medical Corps officer. We had a small medical, dental, and veterinary team. Our medical team extensively used the cheapest parasite medications, pyrantel pamoate and mebendazole, provided by the U.S. Army for about 10,000 Bolivian native Indians.

Before my experience in Bolivia, I used homeopathic and natural parasite remedies with moderate success after detecting disturbances on the large intestine meridian using AMA. I was well aware of hidden parasite problems. When I started using prescribed parasite medications from my experiences in Bolivia to treat irritable bowel syndrome (IBS) patients, I saw dramatic responses that I never expected were possible.

When I began treating patients with intestinal symptoms with prescription parasite medications, some of them told me not only did their IBS get better, but their asthma disappeared, eczema or psoriasis resolved, recurrent pneumonia did not return, chronic fatigue and fibromyalgia got better, anxiety/depression improved, fever of unknown origin went away, migraine headache resolved for the first time in years, brain lesions disappeared on MRIs for some multiple sclerosis (MS) patients, sometimes tumors shrank, and many other medical conditions improved.

I was not treating these conditions, but just treating for parasites based on the disturbance of the large intestine meridian. I was treating them with parasite medications based on 30 years of medical practice and my U.S. Army military experience in Bolivia.

This information was not taught in my medical school or internal medicine training. The **large intestine meridian** is paired with the **lung meridian,** and the paired circuitry of the stomach and spleen meridians. See Figure 3.

Parasites are so pervasive, and yet so difficult to detect by modern medical science. It is not wise to rely exclusively on the standard stool test or blood test to detect parasites. They have a complex lifecycle and many are not confined to the intestinal tract. We need to embrace and understand the concepts of subtle energy fields, matrix, prana, and meridians that have been described in ancient civilizations.

Ayurveda is the oldest existing medical system, having its heritage in ancient India. If Harry Van Gelder's writing, *The Process of Healing*, is correct, the ancient Indian Ayurveda might be the great grandfather of modern homeopathy. According to Van Gelder, Ayurveda mentions three types of medicine for healing: homeopathy, herbs, and drugs.

In Ayurvedic medicine, drugs are only reserved for demonic ("parasites" is my interpretation). I have tried homeopathic and natural herbal parasite remedies with moderate success. But when I used the correct combinations of prescribed parasite medications in the right sequence (in conjunction with resolving hidden dental problems), there were dramatic responses to many unexpected medical conditions that seemed impossible to cure. I am convinced that deeply imbedded parasites manifest in many faces of demonic expression of acute and chronic illnesses. Unlike antibiotics, parasite medications are not covering up symptoms and suppressing the conditions. I am against using medications to cover up symptoms, as promoted by some pharmaceutical companies. I am convinced that parasite medications have been underutilized because parasites are deceptive, shadowy, and demonic. In recent years, Pharma companies have been recognizing the demand for parasite medications and have been aggressively raising prices. They are becoming the monetary parasites on the parasites conundrum.

Figure 3. Large Intestine Meridian

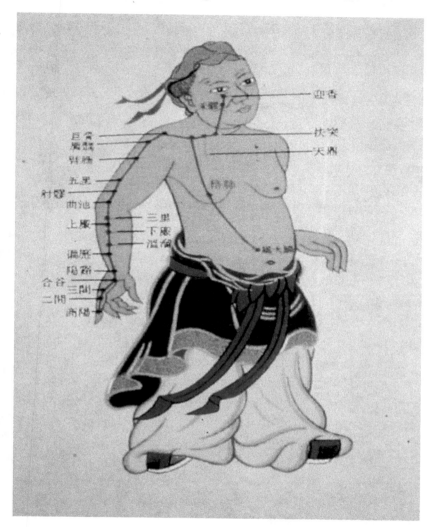

Medical Acupuncture on Dental and Allergy Points

*Look ahead for new discoveries! Dental and allergy points were
not mapped until the 1950s. Seeing a biological dentist or oral
surgeon, and getting medical treatments for heavy metals, toxic
chemicals, and fungal mycotoxins can address these challenges.*

Another lesson I have learned is that there are always new
discoveries ahead. A good example is the **dental and allergy
points**, mapped by Dr. Reinhold Voll of Germany, which give
additional insights into the health of the body and biocybernetics
beyond the meridians discovered by Traditional Chinese Medicine.

A German medical doctor and acupuncturist, Dr. Reinhold Voll,
developed a new meridian system about 60 years ago based on the
classical acupuncture meridian system. He mapped out over 500
acupuncture points that went well beyond the classical system. The
most important of Voll's new classification of the acupuncture
system include the dental/lymph system and allergy meridians, and
other extra meridians including connective/fibroid tissue, joints,
skin/scars, and cellular degeneration points. These points were not
described previously in classical Chinese acupuncture teaching, so
there is no figure to illustrate them. Instead, see Figure 4, the
Tooth-Organ Meridian Chart, in Chapter 6.

In my experience, one of the fastest ways to rebalance the
disturbed acupuncture meridians is by aggressively using parasite
medications (and antifungal medications). The selection of
medications is based on Acupuncture Meridian Assessment.

However, the **dental and allergy meridians** described by Dr. Voll
were often not affected by parasite medications. They seem to be
separate and independent medical problems. I addressed dental-
related medical problems in my first book, *Accidental Cure*, and

they are highlighted here in Chapter 6. Dental problems are a major overlooked factor in many cancers, persistent Lyme cases, chronic diseases, and medically unexplained symptoms (MUS).

The allergy points are another brilliant discovery by Dr. Voll. I like to call them **allergy-immunology points** to reflect their true significance. They reflect both allergy and the immune system. The allergy-immunology points help to unmask not only food and airborne allergies but also hidden toxic metals, environmental toxic chemicals and fungal mycotoxins.

With his educational background as a medical doctor, acupuncturist and homeopathic physician, Dr. Voll was able to diagnose and treat some of the most complex, chronically ill patients. His technique was known as electroacupuncture according to Dr. Voll, or EAV. With modern computer technology, it is called computerized electrodermal screening, or CEDS.

The popularity of EAV and CEDS peaked in the 1970's through 1980's and gradually waned due to the time-consuming complexity of meridian testing based on homeopathic principles, as well as crackdowns on some of the outlandish claims of "cures" by medical, dental and non-medical EAV/CEDS practitioners.

There are current popular systems in use which are based on an artificial intelligence algorithm, not on true meridian assessment. The AI algorithm can predict and prognosticate based on the galvanic currents, age and sex, other proprietary factors derived from blood, urine, saliva, voice analysis, and statistical probability. They claim to predict what kind of medical problems you may have and recommend certain types of treatment plans. This kind of technology is still too young and relatively unknown, and so I do not recommend using this kind of device for medical treatment when you are seriously ill. Instead, stick with the 5,000-year-old disruptive technology called acupuncture and Acupuncture Meridian Assessment.

My experience has demonstrated that the order of treating problems detected by AMA is important. After cleaning out the most common parasites and fungal problems, the next step is to address dental and allergy-immunology related problems.

A deep dental jawbone infection (cavitation) and root canals may have multiple sources of infection, including viruses, bacteria, fungi, parasites and biotoxins, but may not show in up in x-rays. We can gain additional forensic evidence from these subtle energy fields using AMA, and treat the overlooked, sneaky, stealthy, hidden invaders that are asymmetric threats to health.

Part 3
Hidden Invaders: Dental, Fungal and Parasite Conundrum

Chapter 6 Murder by Dentists: A Mouthful of Forensic Evidence

*When the latest
medical therapy fails,
think dental.*

The hardest part of my work is convincing patients to follow up on necessary, sometimes extensive and expensive recommendations for dental work when I find their health problems are likely caused by dental problems. Why are they important? Teeth are integrally connected to the body: through blood supply, lymph, jawbone, gum tissue, and electrical meridian pathways. An infection, a metal or material toxicity reaction, an electrical imbalance, and/or a mechanical problem will manifest in other organs, glands, joints and the like.

Acupuncture Meridian Assessment provides an additional tool to detect links between underlying dental and systemic health problems. As each of the major meridians runs through particular teeth, organs, joints, glands and tissues, a disturbance in the meridian gives an indication – forensic evidence – of where to look for dental problems. My new patient evaluation may also include a panoramic dental x-ray and a head thermography scan. Based on this information, I refer patients to a biological dentist or oral surgeon for needed dental work.

Your teeth and dental problems are rarely included in a medical doctor's diagnostic assessment. This is a tragic consequence of the split between the medical and dental professions. If you have seen many doctors for your condition with an unsuccessful diagnosis, your mouth may be a missing link to your illness.

Dental amalgam, called "silver fillings" for marketing purposes, is actually **50 percent mercury** mixed with other metals. Tiny amounts of mercury off-gas with heat and abrasion over time, in addition to exposure during placement and drilling out old amalgam fillings. Mercury binds tightly to electrons, and toxic levels can build up and accumulate in people who, due to genetic factors, do not methylate (clear heavy metals and toxins) well. Along with root-canal-treated teeth, they serve as asymmetric threats in dental-induced illnesses, and are often major contributors to a wide variety of unexplained symptoms.

Over the years, physicians and dentists have learned to use increasingly sophisticated laboratory, electromagnetic and radiological methods to detect physical problems that are not "in plain sight." X-rays, ultrasound, CT scans, MRIs and PET scans can detect physical abnormalities, cysts, tumors, and the physical manifestations of infection and inflammation. EEGs and EKGs measure brain and heart activity, and nerve conduction tests measure transmission of signals to limbs. We have sequenced the human genome and catalogued a wide range of infectious diseases, vectors and environmental toxins. Given this, why are so many patients facing chronic diseases, and so many challenged by unexplained illnesses? What are we missing?

My practice has been enhanced by learning Acupuncture Meridian Assessment (AMA). This technique combines the art of diagnosis of imbalances along acupuncture meridians with the science of measurement developed by German biological medicine. Heavy metals, chemicals, additives, dental infections and inflammation, and a spectrum of pathogens change the "biological terrain" of the body, including electron flows, cellular metabolism, the microbiome, and more. These changes are overlapping and synergistic, and lead to inflammation and chronic diseases.

Dental-Related Medical Problems

Dental-related medical problems are an unsuspected problem for many patients. Miracles can happen when the dental work is done in the right sequence. Otherwise, it will become an "AcciDental Blow Up" in you as the title of my book suggests, or murder by dentists. Do not jump into dental work without the proper sequence of detox and nutritional support.

Unsuspected Dental/Medical Complex Problems:

- Amalgams, Mercury and Heavy Metals
- Root Canals
- Cavitations
- Galvanic Currents, the Mouth Battery
- Metal Allergies
- Bonding and Composite Materials
- TMJ
- Tongue Tie
- Implants
- Periodontal/Gum Problems
- High Speed Drilling
- Proprioception
- Parasites and Bruxism
- Pleomorphism of Bacteria, Fungi, Protozoa and Parasites

Learning About Dental-Related Medical Problems

Dr. Doug Cook, DDS, was instrumental in teaching and mentoring me about the integral interconnections between teeth, the oral cavity and the body as a whole, and about using energy-based diagnostics as a tool to identify problems and guide treatment. I highly recommend his easy-to-read book, *Rescued by My Dentist*. I first learned EAV from him, and was introduced to the biological dental associations, whose conferences I attended for many years.

An early pioneer in the field, Hal Huggins, DDS, was among the first to bring awareness of the health impacts of mercury dental amalgam, root canals, and implants to the forefront. He learned about amalgam health impacts from Dr. Olympio Pinto, a Brazilian dentist he met at an American Dental Association (ADA) meeting. Huggins studied the 1930s research of noted Canadian dentist Weston Price, DDS, on the dangers of root canals, and later founded a lab that did DNA testing of extracted root-canal-treated teeth and cavitation bone tissue. He has written numerous books, including, *Uninformed Consent: The Hidden Dangers in Dental Care,* with Thomas E. Levy, MD, JD.

There are now many excellent books on biological dentistry, including *Whole Body Dentistry*, by Mark A. Breiner, DDS, *The Holistic Dental Matrix*, by Nicholas J. Meyer, DDS, DNM, and Thomas Levy's new book, *Hidden Epidemic: Silent Oral Infections Cause Most Heart Attacks and Breast Cancers*.

Dentist's Story: Dr. Blanche Grube

Here is my story… I sat up tall in my seat, proud to be wearing the clinic jacket embroidered with the name Dr. Blanche Grube. On the first day of dental school, the professor told us we were about to embark on a learning journey. After four years of dental school education, we were to be granted the right to be called "doctors of the head and neck."

I was filled with pride, the good kind that tells you inside that you have chosen a noble profession. Then the professors proceeded to teach us how to be tooth carpenters. We learned how to fill cavities with mercury dental amalgam, how to perform root canal treatment on infected tooth pulps and pulpotomy (partial root canal filled with amalgam or steel crown) on children, how to crown a tooth with metal or porcelain, how to fabricate a bridge to replace missing teeth, and how to make a denture and how to extract teeth that were not salvageable. We learned how to fix what was broken, but very little if anything was mentioned about how all this carpentry work would affect the rest of the body.

After ten years of carpentry (oops, I mean conventional) dentistry, I met my future mentor, Dr. Hal Huggins. He told the class that we were about to embark on a learning journey. During this journey, I learned how to become what he believed all dentists should be. That was to be not only a tooth carpenter, but to be a true primary care doctor, connecting the head and neck integrally with the human body and its intricate systems, interactions and rhythms.

We now know that the conditions of the mouth determine patients' risk factors for cardiovascular disease, cancer and autoimmune disease. Most of the materials placed by conventional dentists are known to be incredibly toxic to the patient, to our dental staff, and to us as dentists. We are exposed to the second most toxic element on the planet as mercury is second only to plutonium, and we are exposed to nanosized particles that our bodies cannot always get rid of, as the ability to excrete heavy metals varies by genetics and our history of exposures.

We were told that patients get cavities due to their inability to brush and floss properly. No mention was made of how to read blood chemistry tests to see if there are internal factors that would lead to a person getting cavities, no matter how many times a day they brush! We now know that the electromagnetic field that is created by our bodies and surrounds us affects our health daily.

This natural electromagnetic field is distorted by the metals we place in a patient's mouth when they generate galvanic currents.

Acupuncture Meridians Connect Teeth, Organs, Joints, and More in the Body

To understand the relationship between teeth, organs, and joints in the body, and acupuncture meridians running between them, see the Tooth-Organ Meridian Chart in Figure 4 below (view it in color on my website). It illustrates how factors such as mercury dental amalgams, root canals, periodontal infections, jaw infections (cavitations), and bite problems can have systemic impacts on health and healthy functioning throughout the body. Each tooth is linked to a meridian. When dental problems are present, they must be addressed to improve the body's capacity for healing.

Figure 4. Tooth-Organ Meridian Chart (p. 1 of 2)

Upper Teeth — R side = teeth 1–8, L side = teeth 9–16

Tooth	Sense Organs	Joints	Spinal Segments	Vertebrae	Organs	Endocrine Organs	Others
1	Inner Ear	Shoulder Elbow / Hand, Ulnar Foot, Plantar Toes, Sacro-iliac Joint	C8; T1 T5 T6 T7; S1 S2 S3	C7; T1 T5 T6; S1 S2	Heart-R	Pituitary, Ant. Lobe	CNS Psyche
2	Maxillary Sinus	Jaws / Front of Knee	T11; T12; L1	T11; T12; L1	Duodenum	Para-thyroid	Mammary Gland-R
3	Maxillary Sinus	Jaws / Front of Knee	T11; T12; L1	T11; T12; L1	Pancreas; Stomach-R	Thyroid	Mammary Gland-R
4	Ethmoid Cells	Shoulder Elbow / Hand, Radial Foot, Big Toe	C5 C6 C7; T2 T3 T4; L4 L5	C5 C6 C7; T2 T3 T4; L4 L5	Lung-R	Thymus	
5	Ethmoid Cells	Shoulder Elbow / Hand, Radial Foot, Big Toe	C5 C6 C7; T2 T3 T4; L4 L5	C5 C6 C7; T2 T3 T4; L4 L5	Large Intestine-R	Pituitary, Post Lobe	
6	Eye	Hip / Foot	T8; T9; T10	T9; T10	Liver-R; Gall-bladder	Pituitary, Post Lobe	
7	Frontal Sinus	Back of Knee, Sacrococcyx / Foot	L2 L3; S4 S5; Coccyx	L2 L3; S3 S4 S5; Coccyx	Kidney-R	Pineal Gland	
8	Frontal Sinus	Back of Knee, Sacrococcyx / Foot	L2 L3; S4 S5; Coccyx	L2 L3; S3 S4 S5; Coccyx	Bladder-R Urogenital Area	Pineal Gland	
9	Frontal Sinus	Back of Knee, Sacrococcyx / Foot	L2 L3; S4 S5; Coccyx	L2 L3; S3 S4 S5; Coccyx	Bladder-L Urogenital Area	Pineal Gland	
10	Frontal Sinus	Back of Knee, Sacrococcyx / Foot	L2 L3; S4 S5; Coccyx	L2 L3; S3 S4 S5; Coccyx	Kidney-L	Pineal Gland	
11	Eye	Hip / Foot	T8; T9; T10	T9; T10	Liver-L; Bile Ducts -L	Pituitary, Post Lobe -L	
12	Ethmoid Cells	Shoulder Elbow / Hand, Radial Foot, Big Toe	C5 C6 C7; T2 T3 T4; L4 L5	C5 C6 C7; T2 T3 T4; L4 L5	Large Intestine-L	Pituitary, Post Lobe -L	
13	Ethmoid Cells	Shoulder Elbow / Hand, Radial Foot, Big Toe	C5 C6 C7; T2 T3 T4; L4 L5	C5 C6 C7; T2 T3 T4; L4 L5	Lung-L	Thymus	
14	Maxillary Sinus	Jaws / Front of Knee	T11; T12; L1	T11; T12; L1	Stomach-L	Thyroid	Mammary Gland-L
15	Maxillary Sinus	Jaws / Front of Knee	T11; T12; L1	T11; T12; L1	Spleen	Para-thyroid	Mammary Gland-L
16	Inner Ear	Shoulder Elbow / Hand, Ulnar Foot, Plantar Toes, Sacro-iliac Joint	C8; T1 T5 T6 T7; S1 S2 S3	C7; T1 T5 T6; S1 S2	Heart-L	Pituitary, Ant. Lobe	CNS Psyche

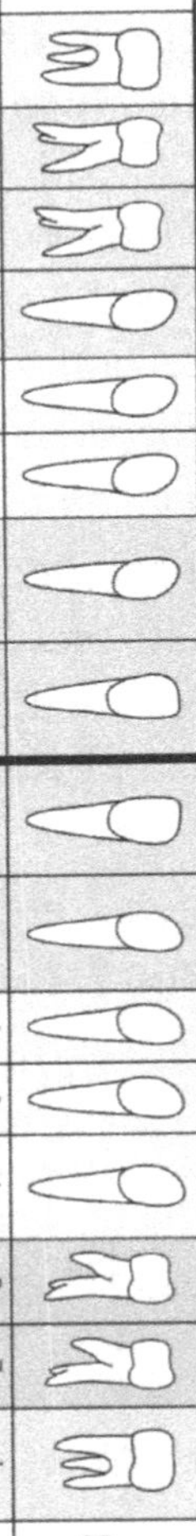

Source: Prevention and Healing, Inc.

Tooth-Organ Meridian Chart (p. 2 of 2)

Lower teeth 17–24 are Left (L); lower teeth 25–32 are Right (R).

Lower Teeth	Others	Endocrine Glands / Tissue System	Organs	Organs	Vertebrae	Spinal Segments	Joints	Joints	Sense Organs
17	Energy Metabolism	Peripheral Nervous System	Jejunum Ileum-L	Heart-L	C7, T1 T5 T6, S1 S2	C8, T1 T5 T6 T7, S1 S2 S3	Shoulder and Elbow		Ear
18		Arteries	Large Intestine-L	Lung-L	C5 C6 C7, T2 T3 T4, L4 L5	C5 C6 C7, T2 T3 T4, L4 L5		Hand, Ulnar Foot, Plantar Toes, Sacro-iliac Joint	
19		Veins	Large Intestine-L	Lung-L	C5 C6 C7, T2 T3 T4, L4 L5	C5 C6 C7, T2 T3 T4, L4 L5		Hand, Radial Foot Big Toe	Ethmoid Cells
20	Mammary Gland-L	Lymph Vessels	Stomach-L	Spleen	T11, T12, L1	T11, T12, L1	Front of Knee	Jaws	Maxillary Sinus
21	Mammary Gland-L		Stomach-L	Spleen	T11, T12, L1	T11, T12, L1	Front of Knee	Jaws	Maxillary Sinus
22		Gonad (Testes or Overy) -L	Bile Ducts -L	Liver-L	T9, T10	T8, T9, T10	Hip		Eye
23		Adrenal Gland	Bladder-L Urogenital Area	Kidney-L	L2 L3, S3 S4 S5, Coccyx	L2 L3, S4 S5, Coccyx	Back of Knee	Foot	Frontal Sinus
24		Adrenal Gland	Bladder-L Urogenital Area	Kidney-L	L2 L3, S3 S4 S5, Coccyx	L2 L3, S4 S5, Coccyx	Sacrococcyx	Foot	Frontal Sinus
25		Adrenal Gland	Bladder-R Urogenital Area	Kidney-R	L2 L3, S3 S4 S5, Coccyx	L2 L3, S4 S5, Coccyx	Sacrococcyx	Foot	Frontal Sinus
26		Adrenal Gland	Bladder-R Urogenital Area	Kidney-R	L2 L3, S3 S4 S5, Coccyx	L2 L3, S4 S5, Coccyx	Back of Knee	Foot	Frontal Sinus
27		Gonad (Testes or Overy)	Gall-bladder	Liver-R	T9, T10	T8, T9, T10	Hip		Eye
28	Mammary Gland-R		Stomach-R Pylorus	Pancreas	T11, T12, L1	T11, T12, L1	Front of Knee	Jaws	Maxillary Sinus
29	Mammary Gland-R	Lymph Vessels	Stomach-R Pylorus	Pancreas	T11, T12, L1	T11, T12, L1	Front of Knee	Jaws	Maxillary Sinus
30		Veins	Large Intestine-R	Lung-R	C5 C6 C7, T2 T3 T4, L4 L5	C5 C6 C7, T2 T3 T4, L4 L5		Hand, Radial Foot Big Toe	Ethmoid Cells
31		Arteries	Large Intestine-R	Lung-R	C5 C6 C7, T2 T3 T4, L4 L5	C5 C6 C7, T2 T3 T4, L4 L5		Hand, Ulnar Foot, Plantar Toes, Sacro-iliac Joint	
32	Energy Metabolism	Peripheral Nerves	Ileum-R, Ileocecal Region	Heart-R	C7, T1 T5 T6, S1 S2	C8, T1 T5 T6 T7, S1 S2 S3	Shoulder and Elbow		Ear

Source: Prevention and Healing, Inc.

Why Are Dental Problems Overlooked in Medicine?

The systemic impacts of oral health are some of the greatest overlooked factors in fueling chronic diseases, including some cancers. Why are they overlooked? There are two major reasons.

First, there is a split, a major disconnect between the dental and medical professions, which leads to ignoring links between diagnosis and treatment of oral and physical health. Second, there is a lot of denial within dentistry that standard practices can cause health problems.

The split is institutionalized: dental care providers, insurance and records are separate from medical care providers, insurance and records. Without considering a patient's dental status, we miss the elephant in the room. Unfortunately, this split is being reproduced, as medical research advances through "Big Data," genomics, immunotherapy, and other developments which do not include patients' dental data.

Second, there is a lot of denial within dentistry that standard practices can cause health problems. The three biggest problems identified by biological dentistry and integrative medicine: mercury dental amalgam fillings cause low-grade mercury poisoning, root canals become infected with biotoxins, and hidden jawbone infections develop years after extraction of wisdom teeth.

In addition, prescreening for biocompatibility of dental materials – which varies by the individual – is required to guide the selection of suitable dental restorative materials. All of these are not only ignored, but denied and suppressed by the mainstream dental profession. As a result, we get into a dental death trap as if "murdered by dentists."

Additional dental causes of health problems which are recognized by the mainstream dental profession include gum disease, electrical currents produced by different metals in the mouth (oral galvanism), and bite problems (malocclusion) including TMJ.

The dental and medical professions are separate and independent of each other. We tend to ignore each other's profession. We seldom communicate and work as a medical-dental team. There is too much "uncertainty" and too wide of a gap for reaching out to other professionals.

I often tell my patients that I will do my part for medical care but the miracle will not happen if you have active hidden dental problems. Dental work must be done properly by a biological dentist or oral surgeon.

Overcoming Resistance to Dental Recommendations

Many of my patients face psychological and financial hurdles to following recommendations for dental work. Psychologically, they have paid dearly for their dental work, and they are afraid of losing teeth. Patients see it as a marker of aging or decline, and they want to keep what they have.

Patients may be more willing to replace a major joint in the body, which is covered by health insurance and requires extensive physical therapy, than to remove root-canal-treated teeth or undertake cavitation (jaw) surgery.

Ironically, an infected root canal or cavitation may lead to degeneration of joints, requiring their replacement, or to a range of chronic diseases and even cancers. A root-canal-treated tooth is a "dead" tooth, and dentistry is the only profession that keeps a dead organ in the body.

Scott's Cavitation Journey

From Better Health Guy's Blog, <u>Cavitation Journey</u>, posted December 2013, updated February 2018.

According to Dr. Louisa Williams, "A cavitation is a cavity or hole of infection in a bone. In surgical nomenclature, cavitation surgery is the term for the dental surgical procedure that removes diseased bone from within this cavity so that new healthy bone can grow back." In my own journey, it was the one thing I had hoped to never have to explore personally, but then if I didn't, I may not get the full Lyme experience (sarcasm).

I shared my first visit with Dr. Simon Yu, MD in my <u>blog</u>. In that consultation, Dr. Yu suggested that there may be a dental issue impacting my overall health. He suspected the most likely was the lower right wisdom tooth extraction site and possibly upper right as well. The minute he said that, I knew he was probably right as lower right had come into question with another practitioner earlier but was not a priority at the time. It was also the site of a dry socket after my wisdom teeth were removed in high school. It seemed clear to me that now was the time I had to address this issue or all of my other efforts to continue to improve my health could be wasted.

I always hoped that I would get through the "Lyme ride" without having to deal with any cavitation work as it had sounded so brutal in the past when I had spoken to others that had done it. That said, I also knew people that found it a very important part of their recovery story. Perry Fields talks about her cavitation experience in her book, *The Tick Slayer*, which I recommend reading.

I went back to St. Louis in late October where I saw Dr. Yu for a follow-up appointment. Overall, his evaluation was much improved after having done a month-long parasite cleanse for a suspected protozoan organism. Surprisingly, even the initial dental stress wasn't as obvious on the second visit, but with enough probing, it was determined to be a likely issue. I worked with Dr. Yu's oral surgeon and had an evaluation to explore it further.

The surgeon indicated that he saw no signs of infection on the panoramic and that my dental health was probably the best that had come through his door. That said, he acknowledged that it would not be the first time Dr. Yu had suggested a possible cavitation that was not visible on X-ray but was found after surgical intervention.

My own muscle testing also suggested that this was an issue that I needed to address, and I knew that if I walked away, I would always wonder if that was a big piece of the puzzle that remained. I kept hearing Dr. Yu say, "If you feel 95% now, you could probably feel 150%," and that there was much potential for even better health. I decided to have the procedure done.

Quite honestly, the anxiety leading up to the procedure was probably worse than the procedure itself. It lasted less than an hour and other than the numbing injections and sensations of pressure, the procedure was very comfortable. When he opened up the sites, the surgeon immediately confirmed that it appeared Dr. Yu was right. The lower right area was "mushy" and as he started to remove bone, it dropped into a hole where the original tooth had been extracted that never filled in with healthy bone. When he opened the upper site, he was surprised by "orange fluid" that started leaking out. After the procedure was complete, I did two days of supportive nutritional IVs.

The recovery was not easy. It took about 8 days before I could remove the gauze from my mouth and eat normally. My cheek had swelled up and apparently was bitten. Thus, when I tried to chew without the gauze, I would bite it again.

For the week after the procedure, I ate mostly smoothies, soups, gluten-free oatmeal, and other soft foods. I had to keep ice on it for several days and then switched to heat. The headband with insertable gel packs made that quite convenient. The only problem was people assumed I had a face lift. I could not fly for 3 days after the procedure and limited any vehicle time as the vibration from driving can dislodge the clot and impact the outcome.

He had given me an Rx pain medication, but fortunately, I didn't even use it. Instead, I used several different homeopathics many times a day. Energetix Dental Chord, Energetix Relief-Tone, and Body Mend were very helpful options. I continue using Dental Chord and will for several months to support the healing process.

The pathology report took several weeks, but ultimately did confirm that both sites were infected. In speaking with other practitioners that have had many patients doing cavitation work, it can be a difficult couple of months afterwards, especially for people that have had Lyme disease as surgeries, accidents, and emotional stress are known triggers that can reactivate infections. Two of my doctors suggested going back on antibiotics if any symptoms were to recur, but these did not appear to be needed with energetic testing, and thus I did not pursue them.

My acupuncturist of several years always found stress in my system, limited energy reserves, and either digestive or kidney weakness. It was a rare day that I would see her that everything looked good. The three visits thus far after the procedure showed a huge shift. She said my body was deeply processing and that my system overall was much stronger. I was honestly blown away by what a difference she was able to sense. She even commented that she was not a supporter of the procedure prior to me having done it, and that I had changed her mind now on cavitation procedures.

A naturopath that I regularly work with for energetic testing usually finds 8-10 new products to either add or rotate in my protocol. After the procedure, there were only two things: one for inflammation which has always been my primary issue and a homeopathic to support the thyroid. I literally thought the fax must not have come through and a page must have been missing! This was another huge validation that things were definitely heading in an even better direction.

I did make a couple of mistakes along the way that I wish I had done differently. I will share them here with the hope that they will help someone in the future.

1) The lab that did the pathology report was disappointing as they made no attempt to identify specific microbes. A practitioner had suggested to me prior to the procedure to get a kit from Dental DNA (now DNA Connexions) and have the sample sent there. I incorrectly believed that the surgeon was familiar with the lab and did not pursue the secondary testing. I now wish I had, as the pathology report was not what I was hoping for.

2) I would have asked for a portion of the sample to make a homeopathic medication from my specific infections. I think this could have been a very powerful healing tool. While it is true that we learn from our mistakes, I hope I never have the opportunity to revisit this kind of a procedure, and that maybe this information will benefit someone else.

Overall, making the decision to address cavitations was the right thing to do. Thanks to Dr. Yu for suggesting I address cavitations, and to the oral surgeon who made it happen. I am grateful.

New Research on Mercury Toxicity from Dental Fillings

The problems with mercury dental amalgam fillings, root canals, and cavitations were outlined in my first book, *Accidental Cure*. There is a lot of information on biological and holistic dentistry on the websites of the International Academy of Oral Medicine and Toxicology (IAOMT), www.iaomt.org, the International Academy of Biological Dentistry and Medicine (IABDM), www.iabdm.org, and the Holistic Dental Association, www.holisticdental.org. See especially the Dental Mercury Facts section of IAOMT's website.

These issues are not well recognized in the U.S., and hotly denied by the American Dental Association (ADA). You may be surprised to learn that other nations have taken the lead in ending dental amalgam use to stop lifelong mercury exposure and reduce environmental impacts. Curiously, ADA affiliates held two patents on dental amalgam. By policy, the AMA does not hold any patents.

Half of U.S. dentists no longer use dental amalgam, and there are now many safer, durable, and more aesthetic alternatives available. Unfortunately, many dental insurance policies favor its use, covering an amount based on the cheaper cost of dental amalgam.

Dental amalgam is now banned in Norway, Sweden, Denmark, Finland, and Japan, and its use is rapidly declining in many other developed and developing nations. Dental amalgam use is to be reduced and phased out under the terms of the Minamata Convention on Mercury, an international treaty to protect human health and the environment which has been ratified by over 100 nations. On July 1, 2018 the European Union's 28 members virtually ended the use of mercury dental amalgam for children under the age of 15 and for pregnant or nursing moms.

Retraction of Findings of Dental Amalgam Safety in the Children's Amalgam Trial

James S. Woods, a University of Washington toxicologist on the original Children's Amalgam Trial team in Portugal, the research study the American Dental Association (ADA) widely cited to show dental amalgam was "safe," was later convinced to reanalyze the data. His team segregated the results by gender and by certain gene types which indicated a reduced methylation pathway. For *boys with four gene types, dental amalgam was associated with neurobehavioral deficits across a range of neurological domains, along with kidney function changes*, over seven years. [12] Lesser effects were associated with another eight genes. Three research papers and a fourth summary article were published 2012-2014.

It is interesting to note that the same impacts were not found in girls. Girls have stronger immune systems and are better able to withstand toxic exposures. As they age and their immune systems weaken, this is likely to change for genetically susceptible women.

Health Impacts on Dentists Exposed to Mercury Dental Amalgam

Thomas R. Duplinsky and Domenic Cicchetti, of the Yale School of Medicine, conducted a study of prescription use by 600 Connecticut dentists compared to a control group matched for gender, age, geographical area, and insurance plan structure. They found *higher rates of neuropsychiatric, neurological, cardiovascular and respiratory disease among Connecticut dentists than carefully matched controls*.[13] They noted, "The greater majority of pediatric and general practice dentists still use mercury dental amalgam restorations. This places them at greater risk than the general population for those disorders, as well as threatening the future health of America's children and adults who continue to receive silver amalgam restorations."

Additional findings on the science and risk of mercury dental amalgam fillings are published on the IAOMT's website, under Dental Mercury Research. You can also search the PubMed database, which has over 28 million citations for biomedical literature from MEDLINE, life science journals and online books.

SMART: Safe Mercury Amalgam Removal Technique

The IAOMT has developed a protocol called the Safe Mercury Amalgam Removal Technique (SMART), which minimizes exposure to mercury vapor during the removal process to the patient, dentist and staff. It is vital to work with a biological dentist for removal of amalgam dental fillings using this protocol, which is explained at www.thesmartchoice.com. Regular high speed drilling, even with a dental dam and copious water spray, increases mercury vapor exposure, and can increase its toxic impact and symptoms.

Root Canal Toxicity

My first book, *Accidental Cure*, described the groundbreaking work of Dr. Weston A. Price, chairman of the American Dental Association 1914-1923, to document serious health impacts of root canals and old tooth extraction sites. One of his most famous experiments was to insert an infected tooth into a series of live rabbits; all died within a couple of weeks. He published a two-volume work of nearly 1,200 pages, later summarized by George Meinig, DDS, in *Root Canal Cover Up,* first published in 1993. This is controversial in the dental profession, given the popularity and prevalence of root canals, so I am sharing new research on the extent of infection and toxicity from root canals below.

New research published in 2018 in the journal *Dentistry* on the relationship between root-canal-treated teeth and systemic disease offers confirmation of the fact that toxins play a part in the disease process.

In the study, German dental researchers Johann Lechner and Volker Von Baehr gathered data from healthy patients and patients with systemic disease: 7 cancer patients, 32 with chronic fatigue and systemic immunological exhaustion, 19 with rheumatoid complaints, 9 with degenerative neurological disease, 18 with atypical facial pain and trigeminal neuralgia, and 12 with intestinal symptoms.

X-rays and cone beam CT scans were taken of each patient's root-canal-treated teeth to look for signs of infection at the root – called apical periodontitis (AP), which can eventually develop into an abscess or cyst. The researchers also measured for sulfur compounds and immunological responses to bacterial toxins.

The study found that ***patients with systemic health problems were up to three times as likely to have infected root canals*** as those in the healthy group: 17.2% versus 5.9%, respectively. Furthermore, some 42.5% "showed immunological disturbance as a result of root-filled teeth."[14]

Based on their findings, the authors found that pathogens in root-canal-treated teeth may indeed raise the risk of systemic health problems. A caveat: The authors concluded, "The data presented here do not prove a cause and effect relation. It could be that the patients demonstrated increased AP due the presence of systemic conditions; an interaction of the systemic conditions vice versa cannot be excluded. Notwithstanding the evidence, the consensus is APs are chronic inflammatory processes and triggering conditions in advance of occurring immune diseases."

Analysis of Root-Canal-Treated Teeth

Boyd Haley, PhD. professor emeritus and former chair of the Department of Chemistry at the University of Kentucky, conducted research on root-canal-treated teeth using today's technology.[15] Studying approximately 900 teeth with root canals for their level of toxicity, he grouped the teeth into three categories:

- 25% of the root-canal-treated teeth had bacteria in them which produced toxins that were fairly benign.
- 50% of the teeth studied contained bacteria that would challenge a healthy immune system.
- 25% of the teeth contained bacteria which produce toxins more powerful than botulinum, widely recognized as the most toxic substance known to humans.

Root canal infections have been implicated in many autoimmune diseases, such as chronic fatigue immune dysfunction syndrome/ myalgic encephalitis (CFIDS/ME) and fibromyalgia, in infectious and environmental diseases such as persistent Lyme and mold and mycotoxin illnesses, in neurological diseases like Amyotrophic Lateral Sclerosis (ALS), Multiple Sclerosis (MS) and Parkinson's Disease, and in certain cancers.

Oral Infections Linked to Brain Pathology, Alzheimer's, Autoimmunity, and Heart Disease

Other infections are implicated in brain pathology. A 2019 study reports that Porphyromonas gingivalis, a key pathogen in gingivitis (gum disease), may be a causative agent in Alzheimer's.[16] A 2016 study of Alzheimer's patients with periodontitis found that infected patients had more rapid cognitive decline.[17] A 2015 paper reported that gum disease was associated with higher amyloid levels in the normal elderly as well.[18] In 2017, infection gum-disease bacteria caused amyloid pathology and cognitive decline in a transgenic mouse model.[19] From my perspective, it is likely not one thing that can trigger or fuel the inflammatory process of Alzheimer's, but many of the legions of asymmetric threats.

Dental and oral infections also play a significant role in autoimmune reactions, as I have found repeatedly in my patients. I am not alone in this. For an explanation with graphic illustrations, see, "The Little Things that Matter: Oral Bacteriophages," by Bonnie Feldman, DDS, MBA, and the slides linked to her post.[20]

Dental and oral infections, as well as mercury toxicity, are also a significant factor in heart disease. Oral infections, dental mercury amalgam, and procedures such as root canals give a double or triple whammy. Jeffrey Dach, MD, debunks the cholesterol myth in his entertaining and easy-to-read, *Heart Book*. Instead of cholesterol, he says to look at endotoxicity from "leaky gut" that causes an inflammatory reaction, lipopolysaccharides (LPS), in the gut lining. What causes leaky gut? The mouth is the gateway to the airway, the gut and the brain.

Towards the end of his book, Dach calls for putting the cholesterol theory of heart disease in the Medical Museum. It has outlived its usefulness, and there is now a much better approach: measuring calcium scores, and limiting inflammation. Perhaps we could also put dental amalgam in the Dental Museum, next to the Golden Mausoleum for Gold Crowns.

Battle Plan: Tom with Squamous Cell Cancer of Thumb

Here is a case study that illustrates how undiagnosed dental problems can synergistically fuel systemic disease and cancer.

Tom, a 53-year-old man came to see me with squamous cell cancer of the right thumb. Acupuncture Meridian Assessment indicated a problem with one of his teeth, even though it looked perfectly normal to the dentist on inspection, including on x-ray. Tom worked as an engineer, and tests indicated a high level of exposure to environmental toxins, including propylene oxide, perchlorate, and mercury. He was highly allergic to buckwheat, garlic, sunflower seeds and walnut, and moderately allergic to lentils and lima beans.

Figure 5 below shows the results of his AMA evaluation, showing a major problem in the dental meridian.

Figure 5. Squamous Cell of Thumb - AMA Evaluation Problem in Dental Meridian

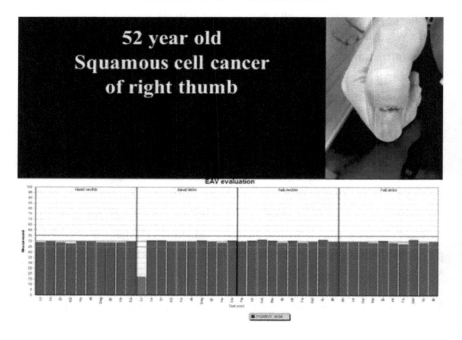

Note: The dental meridian reading is low.

Dental Problems

In Figure 6, the panoramic x-ray is marked to show the abscessed tooth, #11, indicated through further AMA testing. Initially, tooth #10 appeared okay, but subsequent testing revealed a problem there as well. Tom had tooth #11 extracted first, and a year later, followed with an extraction of tooth #10.

Figure 6. Squamous Cell of Thumb - Dental X-Ray
X-Ray Marked with Problem Tooth #11

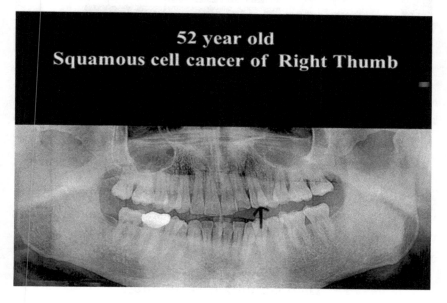

It took some work to convince Tom and his dentist to extract what looked like a perfectly normal tooth, which he did a year later. The specimen was sent to DNA Connexions, a lab that performs polymerase chain reaction (PCR) testing on teeth and jawbone tissue to determine what species of infectious microbes are present. Figure 7 below illustrates the test results of the infections present, followed by an easier-to-read list of the microbes detected.

Figure 7. Squamous Cell of Thumb - DNA Connexions Microbes Detected in Extracted Tooth

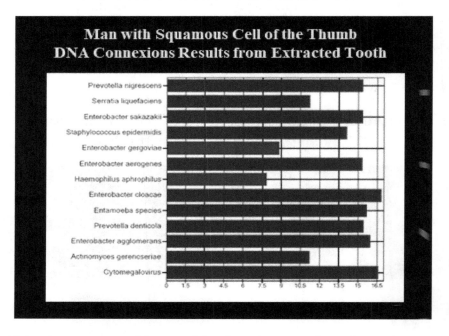

This gives strong evidence of the dental connection – bacteria, viruses, and parasites (Entamoeba is a parasite) – in cancer. Tom's was a complex case which is ongoing, as he had high levels of environmental toxins, and the cancer had spread to other areas.

DNA Connexions Results: List of Microbes Detected

Prevotella nigrescens
Serratia liquefaciens
Enterobacter sakazakii
Staphylococcus epidermis
Enterobacter gergoviae
Enterobacter aerogenes (Klebsiella aerogenes)
Haemophilus aphrophilus

Enterobacter cloacae

Entamoeba species

Prevotella denticola

Enterobacter agglomerans (Pantoea agglomerans)

Actinomyces gerencseriae

Cytomegalovirus

The list gives an indication of how root-canal-treated teeth and/or jawbone cavitations, even when asymptomatic, can harbor long-term infections and help spread systemic disease.

As I wrote in *Accidental Cure*, *"When the latest medical therapy fails, think dental."* Your dental problems can be your death trap! Choose your dentist very carefully.

How to Find a Biological Dentist

There are three associations of biological and holistic dentists in the United States, which also have international members. Each provides a listing of members on its website. Here is their contact information.

International Academy of Oral Medicine and Toxicology
8297 ChampionsGate Blvd, #193 ChampionsGate, FL 33896
(863) 420-6373
Website: www.iaomt.org
Find a dentist: https://iaomt.org/for-patients/search/

International Academy of Biological Dentistry and Medicine
19122 Camellia Bend Circle Spring, Texas 77379
(281) 651-1745
Website: www.iabdm.org
Find a dentist: https://iabdm.org/location/

Holistic Dental Association
1825 Ponce de Leon Blvd. #148 Coral Gables, FL 33134
(305) 356-7338
Website: www.holisticdental.org
Find a dentist: http://holisticdental.org/find-a-holistic-dentist/

Many biological and holistic dentists use the Safe Mercury Amalgam Removal Technique (SMART) developed by IAOMT to protect dental patients, staff, and dentists themselves from exposure to mercury vapor. They are also knowledgeable about screening patients for biocompatibility of dental materials, which as with foods, personal care products, medical devices and environmental exposures, varies by the individual.

Testing options for dental materials biocompatibility include BioComp Laboratories, and Clifford Consulting & Research. In addition, DNA Connexions laboratory tests dental DNA from extracted root-canal-treated teeth, and from jawbone cavitations. Its Oral Panel provides a detailed microbial report using PCR analysis, well beyond a standard pathology report.

Article: Death Certificate for the Unknown Cause: AcciDental Blow Up in Medicine

This article illustrates how dental problems are often overlooked in the development and progression of disease. Why is it so hard to convince patients that an old extracted wisdom tooth jaw can harbor stealthy, deadly, asymmetric threats to health? Also, an amazing story of high blood pressure reversal – my wife!

A request to sign the death certificate for my 65-year-old patient, Sam, whom I had not seen in over two years, arrived on my desk. He lived out of town and apparently had died in his sleep from the probable cause of a cardiovascular event. The mortuary in his town could not find a physician to sign the death certificate, so the family requested me to sign it. He had a history of hypertension, stroke and severe fatigue. Sam always said, "I have zero energy."

Reviewing his chart, Sam used to be a heavy drinker and heavy smoker. He was taking high blood pressure medications and lots of natural, herbal and vitamin supplements recommended by a well-known natural doctor. My notes indicated his underlying problem most likely came from a hidden dental infection in his lower wisdom teeth areas #17 and #32, according to AMA. I recommended he see an oral surgeon.

Sam did not like my evaluation pointing to his jaw-dental area, since all his rotting teeth had been extracted based on my recommendation a few years earlier. Apparently, his dental infection had progressed into his jawbone from his old wisdom tooth area, which corresponded to his heart-energy system according to the organ-meridian-dental chart. See the Tooth-Organ Meridian Chart on my website, or earlier in this chapter. Sam kept reminding me that he had no teeth, so he could not possibly have another dental infection. He was angry at my recommendation for more dental work to be done, and did not come back.

We can easily attribute Sam's heavy smoking and drinking as the cause of his death. There is unfortunately no proof that his dental infection was contributing to his hypertension, stroke and death from the cardiovascular event. There is a disconnection between the dental and medical professions in connecting the dots between causes and effects. Recommending dental work as a medical doctor is one of the sure ways of losing your patients.

Dental-related medical conditions are well known and well documented in medical journal articles and textbooks. Yet, they are difficult to evaluate because medical doctors do not have the proper training, and lack the diagnostic tools to detect dental-related medical problems. Unknowingly, dentists may plant the seed for a "biological time bomb" when they drill or extract a tooth, place amalgams, perform root canals and implants, etc.

Since the time of the Stone Age – about 13,000 years ago – dental infections have been common, and Stone Age people had cavities treated by Stone Age dentists. They did not drill and fill cavities with mercury-containing dental amalgams. They did not use high speed drills or perform root canals or implants. They scraped and coated the cavity with bitumen, a sticky, tarlike substance Stone Age folks used to attach stone tools to handles. This history is brought to you by a team of two biological anthropologists, Oxilia and Benazzi, from the University of Bologna in Italy (*Science News*, May 2017, on *American Journal of Physical Anthropology*).

I have personally experienced significant dental problems. Under mental stress from organizing a conference, one day I woke up with swollen gums/teeth and could barely get out of bed with severe fatigue. That tooth was eventually extracted and no root canal was done. On another occasion, I cracked one of my teeth while eating salad that unknowingly had an olive pit. The tooth got infected and was later extracted. After, I had persistent knee pain lasting over 18 months. If I was one of the Stone Age men with an infected tooth I may have written my own death certificate.

Unrecognized, untreated high blood pressure is considered a leading silent killer, affecting millions of people. I saw a malignant hypertension patient with blood pressure of 250/150. My AMA exam showed surprisingly only a dental problem. I sent the patient to an oral surgeon for a suspected infection at the old wisdom tooth area at #17. The day after oral surgery, her blood pressure was at 140/85. That person happened to be my wife!

Almost every known chronic illness – from arthritis, cardiopulmonary-vascular problems of all kinds, autoimmune disease, kidney problems, neurologic-muscular disorders, gastrointestinal-urological-skin-immunological problems, Lyme-like conditions, and many cancerous conditions – can be associated with unrecognized dental problems. Chronic illnesses can result from use of toxic materials like mercury, nickel or allergenic bonding materials, excessive galvanic currents, and from infected root canals and jawbones (even after tooth extractions).

If you have unexplained chronic medical conditions, consider unrecognized hidden dental problems that may be triggering mysterious unexplained symptoms – despite normal looking dental x-rays. Malignant hypertension or another serious health threat caused by hidden dental problems is not an accident. This condition does not require more blood pressure medications, but a competent dentist or oral surgeon to correct hidden dental problems.

Holistic, biological dental groups understand the dangers of modern dentistry and the dangers of "AcciDental Blow Up in Medicine." When the medical profession recognizes the gravity of the AcciDental Blow Up in Medicine – planted by a dentist many years ago in the dental chair – we should ask the mortuary to send the death certificate to the dentist. For my patient, I filled out the certificate with the immediate cause of death as a cardiovascular event most likely from heart attack due to heavy smoking, hypertension and history of previous stroke. The death certificate did not mention dental infection: the unknown but likely cause.

Article: Murder by Dentists, Saved by Holistic Dental Groups: Tolerating Uncertainty as the Next Medical Revolution

225,000 people each year die from medical care. How many of those deaths start in the dental chair with improper dental care, mercury dental amalgams, root canals, faulty tooth extractions, and other dental-related problems?

Two main American biological dental groups, the International Academy of Oral Medicine and Toxicology (IAOMT) and the International Academy of Biological Dentistry and Medicine (IABDM), had their first joint meeting in Reno, NV in September 2016. These Holistic Dental Groups have been leaders in the Dental-Medical health care reform movement.

They are against using silver-mercury amalgams, conservative in the use of root canals and dental implants, careful in their use of dental materials, and address issues of TMJ (Temporomandibular Joint), jaw infection, sleep apnea, and other dental related medical issues that are not widely accepted by the main stream or academic medical communities.

I had the privilege to present to over 500 biological dentists on "Dental, Parasites and Energy Medicine: Missing Link for Incurables." I discussed how medical professionals can detect problems before they manifest in blood tests or X-rays by using ancient subtle energy medicine, which I call Acupuncture Meridian Assessment (AMA).

One of my lecture slides covered medical related iatrogenic death, that is, death caused by physicians and medical care (225,000 people die every year from medical care, JAMA 2005). But I said it's not fair for medical care to take all the blame for these deaths.

Often the problems started in the dental chair with improper dental care, mercury amalgams, root canals, faulty tooth extractions, and other dental-related problems.

Many books and articles have been written about "death by medical care." I raised the question, "How about murder by dentist?" The audience was dead silent. They did not appreciate my sense of warped sense of humor and counterargument. At least, not until I said that maybe these patients can be saved by holistic dental groups like you.

The dental and medical professions are separate and independent of each other. We tend to ignore each other's profession. We seldom communicate and work as a medical-dental team. There is too much "uncertainty" and too wide of a gap for reaching out to other professionals. I often tell my patients that I will do my part for medical care, but the miracle will not happen if you have active hidden dental problems. Dental work must be done properly by a holistic dentist or oral surgeon.

Dealing with uncertainty in medical science is a familiar, but uncomfortable, territory for medicine and dentistry. In November 2016, the *New England Journal of Medicine* published an essay, "Becoming a Physician; Tolerating Uncertainty – The Next Medical Revolution?" by Arabella L. Simpkin, BM, BCh, MMSc, and Richard M. Schwartzstein, MD.[21]

The essay discussed that, although physicians are rationally aware when uncertainty exists, the culture of medicine is unwilling to acknowledge and embrace uncertainty. They continued that we demand a differential diagnosis after being presented with few facts and exhort our trainees to "put your money down" on a solution to the problem at hand despite the powerful effect of cognitive biases under these conditions.

Great tensions are created by the conflict between the quest for certainty and the reality of uncertainty. Our curricula should recognize diagnosis as dynamic and evolving. We can speak about "hypotheses" rather than "diagnosis," thereby changing the expectations of both patients and physicians and facilitating the shift in culture.

Sir William Osler's (Father of Modern Medicine, one of the founders and professor of Johns Hopkins Hospital) maxims states that medicine is a science of uncertainty and an art of probability. Ironically, only uncertainty is a sure thing. Certainty is an illusion.

Therefore, we can, and should, teach physicians specifically about handling scientific uncertainty, which is essential if patients are to truly share in decision making.

The *New England Journal of Medicine* (NEJM), a conservative medical journal from the Massachusetts Medical Society, is telling physicians to tolerate and teach young physicians to deal with uncertainty as a new reality in this binary black and white, yes and no, digital age.

The basic principle of uncertainty in quantum physics can be applied to all living systems, including medical and dental related biological systems. Based on Acupuncture Meridian Assessment (AMA), I may tell my patients with asthma, heart arrhythmia, chest pain, chronic fatigue, rheumatism, Lyme disease, kidney problems, infertility, or hormonal problems to remove a tooth that may look normal according to X-rays and go through aggressive parasite cleansing. Some patients look at me as if I am too far gone, as if I am pretending to see from the dark side of the moon.

Even when a patient is willing to extract the tooth (with no promise that it will fix their problems), it is very difficult to convince a regular dentist, or even a holistic dentist, to remove the tooth without the hard evidence of an X-ray indicating an abscessed or damaged tooth. The pathological effects of biotoxins from any infected tooth in the early stage of a tooth infection may not manifest on X-ray for many years or until there is over 30-50% damage to the jaw bone. However, the abnormal disturbance signal can be picked up by acupuncture meridian assessment at a much earlier phase of the illness, even before showing physical evidence by X-ray.

Tolerating uncertainty might be the next medical revolution according to the NEJM essay. Murder by dentist, saved by holistic dental groups, may not sound as crazy as murder by medical care. Sometimes, dealing with the dental related medical problems by medical professionals or dentists are like looking blindfolded at the dark side of the moon.

Chapter 7 Parasites as Masters of Deception

Are we at the top of the food chain, or at the bottom? How about both?

To understand the problem of parasites as invaders stealing our health, it helps to step back and look at the great circle of life. All living things evolved from universal ancestors. We coexist with them – and also compete with them.

Universal Ancestors and the Evolution of Life

In the great circle of life and evolutionary biology, our ancestors predate us on the evolutionary time scale, yet continue to live within us and help chart our destiny and health. The three domains of life are:

- Archaea: without a cell nucleus, living in extreme environments,
- Bacteria: single-celled organisms that lack a nucleus but have different cell wall characteristics, and
- Eukaryotes: organisms with a cell nucleus within a membrane.

Eukaryotes vary from single-celled organisms to complex multicellular animals and plants. In fact, most living things are eukaryotes, made up of cells with distinct nuclei and chromosomes that contain their DNA.

The six kingdoms of life include: Archaea, Bacteria, Protists, Fungi, Plant, and Animal. There are symbiotic and parasitic relationships up and down the food chain. In other words, we are not only influenced by what we eat, but by what is eating us. See Figure 8, which instead of putting parasites under humans in the evolutionary (and food) chain moves them upward. Our metabolism and health is influenced by many things, not only what we eat, but what we are feeding and reproducing inside us. Think of the microbiome as a little zoo and fungi habitat which extends beyond the digestive tract.

Figure 8. The Kingdoms of Life
Creation, Evolution and Co-Creation

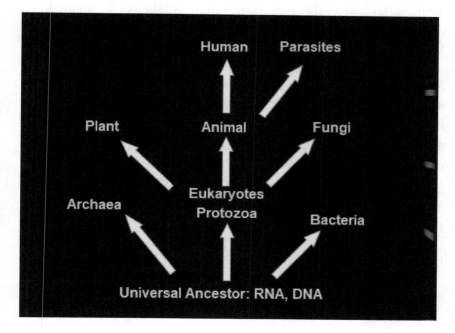

Are we at the top of the food chain, or at the bottom? How about both?

Depending on the health of our biological terrain and the status of our invaders, we can have a peaceable kingdom or a Game of Thrones.

The Parasite Paradox

Why are parasite problems overlooked? They're overlooked because there are no reliable ways to detect parasites, many of them live outside the GI tract, and we assume parasites are only in Third World countries. Also overlooked is the transfer of parasites on a global basis due to worldwide global migration, change in diets around the world, global climate change, and global travel.

Using a U.S. Army military operations analogy, parasites are an asymmetric threat, engaged in unconventional warfare with humans. Unconventional warfare can be conducted by using countermeasures based on Energy Medicine and Acupuncture Meridian Assessment to track, monitor and neutralize them.

Many parasite problems manifest outside of the GI tract, such as asthma or bronchiectasis in the lung, brain fog or migraine headache, anemia, cyst, tumor, allergies or suppression of allergies, chronic fatigue and fibromyalgia, behavioral or vision problems, etc. Another strategy is thinking of parasites and parasitic infectious relationships. Parasites have their own associated concurrent co-infections with viruses, bacteria, and fungi.

Figure 9 shows the transmission lifecycle of the liver fluke.

Figure 9. Lifecycle of Liver Fluke
(Fasciola hepatica)

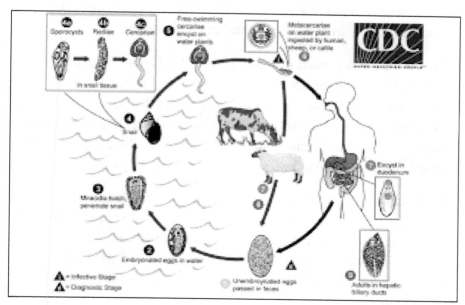

Source: Centers for Disease Control and Prevention, **Fasciola Biology** https://www.cdc.gov/parasites/fasciola/biology.html.

A global medical literature review by Florian H. Pilsczek of the University of Calgary, Canada found 21 articles reporting 68 cases of parasites mimicking malignancies, such as spinal cord tumors by Angiostrongylus, lung cancer by Strongyloides stercoralis and Paragonimus westermani, brain tumor by Schistosoma, colon tumor by Fasciola hepatica, and duodenum adenoma carcinoma by Strongyloides stercoralis.[22]

A review by Vassilis Samaras et al. in *The Journal of Infection in Developing Countries* also showed a connection between chronic bacterial and parasitic infections and cancer, such as Salmonella typhi with carcinoma of gallbladder and pancreas, chlamydia with carcinoma of lung, ovary, and lymphoma, Schistosoma with bladder, cervical, colorectal, and liver cancer, liver flukes with cholangiocarcinoma, and chronic osteomyelitis with myeloma, fibrosarcoma, and angiosarcoma.[23] The most common source of osteomyelitis is from hidden dental/jaw infections.

One of the hardest parts of treating parasites is that there are no reliable tests available. Several of my articles have addressed the shortcomings in using stool tests. Stool tests miss parasites in other parts of the body, such as the brain, kidneys, liver, lungs, pancreas and more. Stool tests can also miss them in the GI tract due to sample size, and due to parasites' lifecycles in the body.

Veterinarians are familiar with parasite problems in animals. They routinely prescribe parasite medications. But medical professionals are afraid to treat parasites unless we can identify the type of parasite. They do not initiate routine parasite medications even when they highly suspect that patients might be suffering from parasite infestations.

Regular deworming and routine dental care have doubled the average life span of horses, according to a patient who is a professional horse breeder. Can you imagine doubling the human life span by routine deworming and dental care? That would be an absolute nightmare for the government! Anti-aging medical doctors may need to know how to use parasite medications if they are serious about prevention, healing and longevity medicine.

Types of Parasites

In the United States, the most common human parasites are microscopic protozoa (single cell, amoeba-like) that can be transmitted by air, food, water, insects, animals, and other humans. The most common protozoal parasites are Giardia lamblia, Entamoeba histolytica, Dientamoeba fragilis, and

Cryptosporidium. Other types of parasites include pinworms, roundworms, tapeworms, Trichinella spiralis, hookworms and filaria. See Figure 10, which illustrates the Human Parasites' Family Tree.

Figure 10. Human Parasites' Family Tree Protozoa and Metazoa

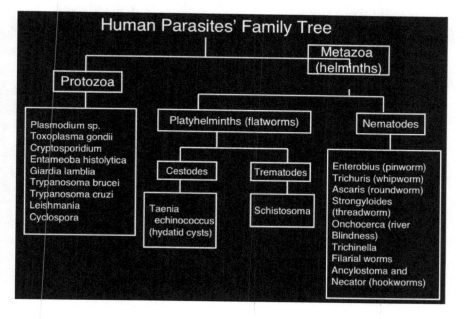

Source: Darvin Scott Smith, MSc, MD, Stanford University

Patient Perspective on Parasites: Misery Loves Company

When it comes to parasite problems, many patients have multiple infections. Having one kind may invite others and make conditions more hospitable for them. One of my patients said when it comes to parasites, misery loves company. Parasites remind her of cousins – they get together and invite others to join them and have a party. "Hey, come in, let's meet here!" In addition, bacteria, and even parasites, can bring their own parasites, as the Lyme spirochete can be accompanied by Bartonella, Babesia, Ehrlichia, or Anaplasma. This is one of the reasons that simultaneous, concurrent treatment by different medications is indicated.

Parasites and Allergies: Similarity of Symptoms

I have compiled common symptoms associated with parasite infection and allergy-related problems. You may be surprised to see the similarity of symptoms. Many symptoms that indicate a parasite infestation also indicate allergy problems and vice versa, as shown in the matching columns in the first grouping in Table 1 below. The columns in the second grouping don't match, but can influence one another, as if parasite and allergy symptoms were running a parallel course.

Note: There is a crossover article on Parasites and Meat Allergies (from a tick-borne parasite) at the end of this chapter.

Table 1. Comparing Parasite and Allergy Symptoms

Parasites	Allergies
Common Symptoms	**Common Symptoms**
Asthma	Asthma
Bloating	Bloating
Brain fog	Brain fog
Cramps	Cramps
Diarrhea	Diarrhea
Fatigue	Fatigue
Flatulence	Flatulence
Gallbladder attack	Gallbladder attack
Headaches	Headaches
Immune deficiency	Immune dysfunction
Irritable bowel syndrome	Irritable bowel syndrome
Mucous secretion	Mucous secretion
Muscle problems	Muscle pain
Ulcerative colitis	Ulcerative colitis
Weight gain	Weight gain
Weight loss	Weight loss
Parasites	**Allergies**
Different Symptoms	**Different Symptoms**
Anal itching	Abdominal pain
Appendicitis	Acne
Brain abscess	ADD/ADHD
Cancer	Anorexia
Cardiomyopathy	Bedwetting
Constipation	Behavioral changes
Coughs	Bronchitis
Dermatitis	Canker sores
Eczema	Celiac disease

Fever	Conjunctivitis
General pain	Ear Infection
Hallucination	Edema
Indigestion	Hives
Inflammations	Hypoglycemia
Insomnia	Irregular heartbeat
Intestinal bleeding	Irritability
Liver dysfunction	Itching
Mal-absorption	Joint pain
Memory loss	Low back pain
Nausea	Seizures
Peritonitis	Sinusitis
Poor coordination	Skin rash
Pulmonary fibrosis	Urinary problems
Urogenital dysfunctions	Urticaria (hives)

Treating Parasite Infections

I have included a special Chapter 12 later in this book, "Parasite Medication Guidelines for Physicians," which outlines protocols for treatment of different kinds of parasite infections with a variety of prescription drugs, including drug combinations and sequences when persistent infections indicate. My first book, *Accidental Cure*, contains additional information on treating parasite infections, including herbs and supplements which may be helpful. In my experience, for persistent infections, prescription medications are required – and often yield surprising health benefits.

Below is a blog post from one of my patients, and some of my favorite articles on parasites, their challenges, and how to detect and treat them. There are many more articles on my website, listed on my Articles page.

Scott's Blog: Simon Who? Yes, That's Right. Simon Yu

From Better Health Guy's Blog, "Simon Who? Yes, That's Right. Simon Yu MD," on parasite treatment posted September 2013.

Overall, I've done well with my recovery and often feel I've reached 95%. I continue to look for other tools to lead to even better health. I still have inflammation, especially in my upper shoulders and neck, which I would like to reduce.

I wanted to support my immune response, and I just seem to be more prone to inflammation than I want to be. So, I made the trip to St. Louis, Missouri to work with Dr. Simon Yu, MD.

I read Dr. Yu's book *Accidental Cure* a few years ago when it first came out. I've met him at a couple of conferences in the past. I've done some of his protocols through my work with another doctor, but I never had the opportunity to see him myself. He was hosting a conference in September 2013 near his office. I called to see if he had an opening the day before the event, and the universe gifted me the opportunity to see him. I was there from 9 am until after 4pm. What a day it was!

Dr. Yu uses many different tools and techniques and is a skilled master in pinpointing potential causes of "dis-ease." Two of his specialties are the treatment of parasites which is described in detail in his book and the impact of dental issues on health.

A number of different energetic testing modalities are used in an appointment including the use of a Mora device to look for stress in various meridians. He measures of total of 40 points and makes the analogy that each point is like a string on a violin. Any of them can be out of tune. In my case, 8 out of 40 were "out of tune" and indicated some opportunity for improvement. Once he has run through all of these points, he literally plays the meridian points like a piano and listens to what they tell him.

In my case, here's what he felt were areas where improvements might be made:

Heavy metals were a theme and came up several times in our discussion. They seemed to be causing allergies and thyroid stress. In fact, I seemed to have an allergic reaction to the heavy metals themselves.

A protozoan parasite was adding stress to my adrenals and triple warmer meridian which is involved in hormone balance.

Dental infection in one, possibly two, wisdom tooth sites appeared to be an issue. Interestingly, the one site that he said was the most likely to be problematic was the one where I had a dry socket after wisdom tooth removal in high school. I hadn't told him anything about that until after he pinpointed it. This had come up in the past with one other practitioner but at the time did not seem to be a consistent or priority issue. Looks like it may be coming to the top of the list. He suggested that there appeared to be a mixed infection in the old extraction site; likely dental spirochetes.

Those were the main findings. The next 30 days consisted of another round of parasite cleansing with ivermectin, Biltricide, and MediHerb Wormwood Complex along with a homeopathic for allergy and detoxification. I also started Double Helix Water which I've tried in the past but seeing it clearly have an effect on the meridians on the Mora is enough for me to revisit it.

He also did thermography which showed no obvious issues. Hair analysis was done along with a DMPS-provoked metal test for heavy metals. Blood was drawn for food allergies. I've had some of these done in the past, but Dr. Yu has his ways of doing these and I decided to do them again to see what other information they reveal.

Overall, I was impressed by Dr. Yu and felt that he was a very compassionate doctor that brings some very unique skills to the table. I'm looking forward to continuing to explore the issues that he identified in our appointment. As he said, if I feel 95% today, I haven't realized yet how good I can feel. That's a good thought...

Article: Parasites Speak Many Languages

Many people think of parasites in the developing world. However, they are global in scale and can afflict people everywhere. There are more parasites and greater diversity of species than all mammals, reptiles, birds and fish combined. Many have them! We cannot control parasites without retraining medical professionals.

Have you met any parasitologists, scientists who study parasites? They don't usually get the same respect as most scientists. Maybe it's because parasitologists are people who get more excited seeing alien critters or reptiles and dissecting their guts and analyzing the feces rather than seeing a human in a remote island. However, the work they do can produce amazing insights applicable to humans.

I had met only one parasitologist in my medical career until I attended my first parasitology conference, the 84th Annual Meeting of the American Society of Parasitologists. Hundreds of parasitologists from all over the world shared the latest information on parasites from lifecycles, epidemiology, physiology, chemotherapy, genomics, molecular biology, immunology, ecology, and evolutionary biology. They are biologists, veterinarians, and hard core scientists from universities and government agencies. Noticeably absent were medical doctors. In fact, I didn't meet a single medical doctor at the conference.

One of the main themes of the conference was, "Parasites on a Shrinking Planet." Parasites, not viruses, are the leading cause of premature death in the world. One of the most well-known illnesses caused by a parasite is malaria. The parasite is often transmitted by mosquitoes. Another common class of infections and diseases are schistosomiases which are caused by Schistosoma, a genus of parasites.

There has been more public and media attention on viral infections, such as influenza flu, avian flu or swine flu, than of parasites. We've been led to believe that parasites are only in tropical countries like Africa, Mexico, India, South America or Southeast Asia and not an imminent threat in the U.S.

The U.S. government considers any viral epidemic infection as a potential biological-medical terrorism candidate and threat to national and global security. Therefore, the federal government and pharmaceutical companies are racing to develop vaccines for swine flu and influenza flu. However, parasites may be a greater threat as an influencing factor in many common and chronic illnesses.

Parasites have evolved from the beginning of life. There are more parasites and greater diversity of parasite species than all mammals, reptiles, birds and fish combined. Parasites are one of the dominant forces in the evolutionary biology of living systems. Although not commonly expected, parasites are actually quite common in "developed" countries, and in cosmopolitan cities such as New York City, Los Angeles, San Francisco, London, Paris and Amsterdam.

Parasites may also play a very important role in susceptibility to co-infections from viruses. There has been intense study on Schistosoma's role, as well as the malaria parasite's role, in the prevalence of HIV co-infection in Africa.

Global warming, environmental pollution, overpopulation, and the increase in the speed of human activity and human migrations around the world have all had profound impacts on emerging infectious diseases and unrecognized medical problems. Medical doctors are not fully aware of the clinical implications of emerging parasite migrations into new territories due to incredibly mobile global populations.

Many new unexplainable chronic conditions such as fibromyalgia, chronic fatigue, autoimmune disease, cardiovascular disease and cancer are influenced by the cumulative effects of environmental toxins, improper diets, nutritional deficiencies, undetected dental infections, and hidden parasites.

My combined experience in Bolivia during my military reserve duty in 2001 and my observance of extremely chronically ill patients without definite diagnoses has convinced me that almost everyone has parasites. That may sound like an exaggeration. However, the illnesses in which parasites may be causative factors are extensive.

We cannot control parasites without changing the basic social structures, water and food supplies, and general sanitation, and without retraining medical professionals. We are dealing with new parasites, as well as older reemerging parasites that have been neglected for many decades because we thought these common parasites had been eradicated.

Article: Big Whack Theory: Invasion of Parasites, Bacteria, Virus, and Fungus

Physicians ask why I use such high doses of parasite medications for such a long period of time. Higher doses of combinations of parasite medications often give fewer side effects. Per U.S. Army doctrine, "Superior fire power is the best preventive medicine."

Have you ever heard of the Big Whack theory? Most people have heard of the Big Bang theory to explain the creation of the universe 13.8 billion years ago. The Big Bang theory was developed in 1929 based on Edwin Hubble's observation that the distance far-away galaxies were moving away from each other was strongly correlated with their Doppler redshifts. It has been a darling scientific achievement, widely accepted within the scientific community and by the public.

George Lemaitre, a Belgian physicist and Roman Catholic priest, first proposed what became the Big Bang theory. Hubble proved Lemaitre's theory and Hubble got the credit with Hubble's Law about the expansion of the universe. The Hubble telescope was named after him.

But, what is the Big Whack theory? It is a new theory developed in the 1970s to explain the origin of the Moon. The Big Whack theory has never been widely known or acknowledged within the scientific community or by the public, while the Big Bang theory has been taught at school as a matter of fact.

On September 25, 1997, the Los Angeles Times science section covered the story of the Big Whack theory of how the Moon was formed. This leading theory of how the moon was created explains that in a powerful collision, dubbed the "Big Whack," about 4.5 billion years ago, an object more massive than Mars slammed into the infant Earth so hard that its iron core plunged to the center of our planet.

Some of this rock, the theory goes, went skittering into orbits as extremely hot vapor and other debris. Eventually, the vapor cooled and condensed into a spinning disk and eventually clumped up to form the moon in a very short period of time, as little as a year.

For every theory, there are counterarguments. How can one explain the time before the Big Bang? The Big Bang was preceded by a Big Crunch, another theory, and the universe endlessly cycles from one process to the other. Roger Penrose of Oxford states that the Big Bang, in which the visible universe began, was not actually the beginning of everything that we know of as our universe. It was merely the latest example of a series of such bangs that renew reality when it is getting tired out. He thinks that the pre-Big-Bang past has left an imprint on the present that can be detected and analyzed. For more detail, you may read my article in Chapter 2, "Disappearance of the Universe as We Know It for WIMPS: What If Cancer Patient Doesn't Really Have Cancer?"

Why am I bringing up the Big Whack theory and the Big Bang theory? The Big Whack theory may sound more amusing but it has more scientific evidence than the Big Bang theory. Even more fascinating is that the Big Whack theory was already documented several thousand years ago in Sumerian clay tablets. Zecharia Sitchin, a Russian Jewish scholar who can read ancient Hebrew, Sumerian, and Akkadian, translated the Sumerian clay texts in his book, *The 12th Planet*, offering the explanation of the solar system. How is it possible that ancient Sumerians already knew what modern scientists are just figuring out about our solar system? You can explore by reading his book, *The 12th Planet*.

I have my own idea of the Big Whack theory. It's not about our solar system but how to treat parasites. When I give a lecture on parasites and how to treat them, physicians ask why I use such high doses of parasite medications for such a long period of time. Their patients may have had lots of side effects with much smaller doses, so they are reluctant to give the higher doses I recommend.

One of the biggest mistakes using the dose based on the *Physicians' Desk Reference* (PDR) is that it may not be a lethal dose to kill the parasites. Partially-injured parasites start moving around the body looking for a safe place to hide, like the pancreas, and cause much greater side effects unless you give a high lethal dose to kill them. I call the idea the Big Whack theory on parasites which is based on my own empirical experiences during my U.S. Army peacekeeping mission in Bolivia in 2001.

Higher doses of combinations of parasite medications often give fewer side effects than using lower doses or fewer medications. The U.S. Army Combat Casualty Care Course (C4) dictates that, "Superior fire power is the best preventive medicine." If you use a lower dose of parasite medications, you might be engaged in a Whack-a-mole game of never-ending hide and seek.

Parasites are global problems, spreading and engaged in an asymmetric warfare against mankind. We need to solve parasite problems with an unconventional approach: Acupuncture Meridian Assessment based on biophysics. It is important to understand why we are overlooking parasite problems, and to by understand the environmental toxins and biological terrain that promote parasites to grow and spread.

The ultimate goal is prevention before parasites become out of control. Parasites are already manifesting in many unrecognized hidden epidemic health problems, and only a few physicians are aware of the situation. When you can track, monitor, and get rid of parasites with a big whack using high doses of parasite medications, it is so much easier to control bacterial, viral, and fungal problems that accompany parasites. This is my Big Whack theory on the invasion of parasites, bacteria, viruses, and fungi.

Article: Parasite Treatment Hacked by an MIT Engineer: Think Small, Dream Big for Pandemic

What would you do if I told you that you might be able to treat parasite problems by yourself, without visiting a medical doctor? One of my former patients, an MIT PhD Engineer named Susan L., developed a website to help guide people based on her experience.

What would you do if I told you that you can treat parasite problems by yourself, and treat your family without visiting a medical doctor? It is not simple, but apparently it can be done. I just found out from one of my patients, whom I will call John.

I was driving with my wife, Kate, on my way to the West Coast in January 2017 in my convertible, and became snowbound when several feet of snow fell in Northern Arizona. I did not expect or prepare for a snowstorm on this trip. My wife was not happy with my lack of planning, driving through a snowstorm with summer tires. Luckily, John knew we were driving through, and offered us an invitation to stay at his house for temporary shelter from the storm. My wife said yes, and I did not dare to say no.

We stayed at his house for two nights until we could drive again. John and his wife were gracious hosts, and we had many interesting conversations on worldly topics of medicine, politics, science, religion, etc. During our evening conversation, he got an urgent message from a friend to check out a website on how to treat parasites developed by an MIT engineer.

We went to the website, *Debug Your Health*, developed by Susan L., PhD, from MIT. She lives in California. I almost fell off from my chair. She was my patient, and I had taken care of her and her family a few years ago. Her website extensively covered how to detect hidden parasites and dental-related problems. She is an MIT engineer who cracked the secret of hidden parasites and dental problems based on her experiences as my patient, observing my AMA testing, and from her work with other practitioners. She refined my technique with some form of self-muscle testing.

It took me many years of training in medical school, Internal Medicine training, U.S. Army military medical doctor experiences, and years of trial and error in the clinic to figure out hidden parasite and dental problems. Most medical professionals miss the connections between hidden parasites and dental problems that can impact chronically ill patients. And yet, in a few years, an MIT engineer had figured out how to test for hidden parasites and dental problems based on her personal experiences as my patient, and she was able to "hack" the medical system.

I did not review all of her website, but it is well organized, and worthwhile to explore when you cannot get any help from your medical doctors. I do not necessarily endorse her method of bypassing the medical system, but she seems passionate that she and her family suffered unnecessarily from the lack of understanding in the medical community about hidden parasites and dental problems.

She figured out and cracked the code like a good engineer. I have been pondering her audacity to educate the public and put this information out on the Internet while most physicians are in denial about the existence of parasite and dental problems. There is always the danger of self-treating with the wrong medications by the public, and most medical doctors are not familiar enough with parasite medications to guide these desperate patients.

I like to think small. I treat one patient at a time based on Acupuncture Meridian Assessment. From now on, I can think small and still dream big. I will let engineers think big, dream big, and solve the mystery of pandemic parasite problems: a global environmental health threat. The pandemic is here. The CDC and medical communities are not ready to crack the hidden code for detecting hidden parasites and dental problems. The paradigm is shifting. Dream big and you can hack the medical system by navigating sites such as www.debugyourhealth.com. You may stumble onto an accidental cure, but be mindful of your limitations.

Article: Parasite Infections are Leading to Undiagnosed Health Problems for Veterans

Steve, a Vietnam veteran, had parasite problems for decades. I treated him with antiparasitic and antifungal medications. He shared an article about extensive parasite problems of veterans – toxic hitchhikers from war zones. We owe Vets proper treatment.

In February 2017, I saw Steve, a 69-year-old Vietnam veteran from Asheville, North Carolina with a high suspicion for parasite infection. He was told by his doctor that he has Blastocystis hominis and other undefined and unidentifiable parasites based on stool testing. The doctor didn't know what to do for these undefined parasites. The patient said he was a medical corpsman, U.S. Army infantry in the jungle and exposed to Agent Orange during the Vietnam War.

Steve began to have symptoms two years after returning home, around 1973, with extreme fatigue, abdominal discomfort and pain, diarrhea and constipation, anal itching, varicose veins up to his combat-boot-level in his legs, severe insomnia, hypertension, low testosterone, esophageal spasm, social interaction issues, eye problems, joint pain and periodontal disease.

His physical exam was unremarkable. Acupuncture Meridian Assessment indicated four out of 40 meridians were out of balance.

Liver, spleen and two allergy-immunology points at his left and right hands were out of balance. His liver meridian was balanced with praziquantel, indicating he had been exposed to liver flukes. His spleen meridian was balanced with tinidazole, indicating he may have microscopic protozoan parasites. Allergy-immunology points were balanced with itraconazole and fluconazole, indicating molds and yeast/candida problems.

Steve may or may not have been exposed to these fungi and parasites in the jungle in Vietnam. There is no proof where he got these infections. You do not have to leave Missouri, Iowa or Kansas to get parasites or fungus. I wrote many articles on these subjects including, "Operation Enduring Freedom: Saving Colonel H." and "Parasite Guy on UFO and FUO." Patients usually respond to antiparasitic and antifungal medications. He will be on antiparasitic meds for three weeks, followed by a three-week course of antifungal meds, and he may repeat this cycle 2-3 times.

Steve gave me an article written by Claudia Gary: "Toxic Hitchhikers, Parasites from War Zones."[24] This article discussed parasites and diseases of Southeast Asia – most of which are unknown to American physicians – which have long worried Vietnam Veterans of America (VVA).

Gary's article noted that veterans of all wars must contend with exotic parasites. Parasite infections are one focus of Tropical Medicine, an Infectious Disease subspecialty with a history intertwined with war and British colonization. Some of these infections – such as leishmaniasis, lymphatic filariasis, schistosomiasis and soil-contaminated helminth infections – are termed "neglected tropical diseases."

Two of the most devastating and lasting parasitic infections Vietnam veterans have suffered from are those caused by mosquito-borne filarial worms and foodborne liver flukes. Liver fluke infection can go virtually undetected for decades and then cause a deadly cancer, cholangiocarcinoma.

According to the VA's Veterans Health Initiative, veterans who returned from Iraq are at risk of sand fly fever, malaria, amoebic dysentery, giardiasis, and leishmaniasis. Those who have returned from Afghanistan are at risk of protozoan parasites, Entamoeba histolytica, Giardia lamblia, and soil-transmitted helminths.

Tom Berger, the executive director of VVA's Veterans Health Council, responded to Claudia Gary's article that parasites are one of the major health issues affecting people who have served in the U.S. military, primarily because parasitic infections are so commonly misdiagnosed.

Parasites can have a direct and profound effect on one's emotions and intellectual capacity. They can be the direct cause of depression, irritability, emotional swings, confusion, inability to concentrate, and restlessness. They have many indirect causes as well. Insomnia and broken sleep create fatigue that, in turn, affect most aspects of your life and can lead to difficulties in relationships and overall quality of life.

Tom Berger's final comment was that it is important to talk with your healthcare provider about your military service, particularly about where and when you served, and ask whether you should be screened for parasites. At least he is acknowledging that parasites are common among veterans in the Vietnam War and other war zones as a leading undiagnosed health problem. The only problem is that the screening tests for parasites are not reliable, and they are often still misdiagnosed, undiagnosed and untreated.

After this experience, I realized I need to actively reach out to veterans who are suffering from undiagnosed parasite-related health problems. Parasite testing is not reliable and not treated properly at VA hospitals. This is not unique to VA hospitals. Parasites are commonly hidden from standard diagnostic testing and wait to come out when you are most vulnerable. I seek to reach out to VA hospital physicians, and train their physicians to detect and treat parasites based on Acupuncture Meridian Assessment.

Article: Parasites and a Mystery Disease: Unusual Case from Sweden

There is a small network of ordinary people suffering from parasite problems, outcast, abandoned by the traditional medical community. They find and support each other through the Internet. Ingrid felt she was dying, flew from Sweden to Kentucky, and drove to St. Louis with help from an adopted network of family.

Many of us have parasite problems during our lifetimes, whether we live in California, Missouri, Africa, Australia, India, China or Sweden. I just saw Ingrid, a 24-year-old woman from Stockholm, Sweden with parasite problems. She was banned by the Swedish Emergency Medical department after eight ER visits for unexplainable weird medical and neurological symptoms.

Ingrid had partial facial paralysis with a right face droop, difficulty walking, severe fatigue, heart pain, constipation/diarrhea, bloating, and crawling sensations on her skin after she had HPV vaccination in Sweden at age 20. Initially, doctors thought she might have multiple sclerosis (MS), but later ruled it out. She was told to see a psychiatrist for psychiatric evaluation.

There is a small network of ordinary people suffering from parasite problems, outcast, and abandoned by the traditional medical community. They find and support each other through the Internet. Ingrid felt she was dying, flew from Sweden to Kentucky, and drove to St. Louis with financial help from an adopted network of family, led by a former IBM IT engineer. They are like an underground, clandestine support group, and explore treatments through unconventional means when nothing else has worked.

Ingrid had already been treated with two parasite medications for a few days, and her skin had returned from gray back to normal. Because she had already been treated with medications, I initially could not detect parasite movement. I had to use a more advanced "enhanced interrogation technique" based on Acupuncture Meridian Assessment to unmask parasites deeply embedded in the large intestine, small intestine, liver, and gallbladder meridians. She was put on a trial of parasite medications, ivermectin and praziquantel, for two rounds, without any promises or guarantee for the outcome. Her neurological symptoms were coming from a disturbance of the gallbladder meridian. Refer to my article in Chapter 5, "Medical Acupuncture on Gallbladder Meridian: Therapeutic Illusion of IBS and Autism." She returned to Sweden, and I hope she got better.

The evolution of parasitic relationships is another interesting topic. Parasites have their own groups of parasites in turn, which have been adapting to the rapidly changing modern toxic environment, and evolving at a faster rate than we can adapt. Parasites bring protozoa, intracellular parasites, bacteria, viruses, and fungi. They also serve as hosts, and create their own parasitic relationships both up and down the "food chain." They have become the top of the food chain, not us.

Article: Parasites and Meat Allergies

Could red meat allergies be connected to parasites? Yes, through a tick-borne trigger that has a delayed Immunoglobulin E (IgE) antibody reaction! This article explores the surprising connection: an unintended consequence of altered immune response.

Allergy to red meat is rare, but the incidence is rising, recognized by astute allergists. If you have an allergy, your immune system overreacts to an allergen by producing antibodies called Immunoglobulin E (IgE). A recent journal article on meat allergy by Wilson et al. suggests unexpected IgE-mediated delayed-hypersensitivity to ingested animal products is an increasingly important form of unrecognized food allergy.[25] Typically, IgE allergic response is immediate, not a delayed response.

Meat allergy was first recognized in the 1990's and formally described in 2009. Meat allergy was overlooked by primary care physicians because it does not fall under our understanding of typical allergic reactions. Delayed anaphylaxis to red meat occurs in patients with IgE antibodies against the complex sugar called galactose-alpha-1, 3 galactose (alpha-gal) in the meat.

Investigations have revealed an association between IgE to alpha-gal and tick bites. A Swedish study showed the intestinal tract of the tick (Ixodes ricinus) was positive for mono- and polyclonal antibody against alpha-gal stains. When an infected tick bites, we get exposed to alpha-gal. We react in an unusual delayed anaphylaxis, after several hours, by IgE mediated allergic reaction.

The missing link that has not been clearly explained is why and how tick bites are associated with red meat allergy, when it used to be such a rare event. Investigative journalist Velasquez-Manoff unraveled why some tick bites suddenly caused a strange reaction in susceptible people who eat beef, pork and lamb, in "What the

Mystery of the Tick-Borne Meat Allergy Could Reveal," published in the July 29, 2018 issue of *New York Times Magazine*.[26]

Red meat allergy patients tend to come from the Southeast, and the geographical distribution of cases matched that of a tick-borne disease called Rocky Mountain spotted fever. Patients suffered stomach pain and rashes hours after eating meat, and developed antibodies to alpha-gal. About 80 percent reported a history of strong reaction to tick bites before developing meat allergy.

Australian allergist Sheryl van Nunen described 24 cases of meat allergy associated with tick bites in 2007, and nobody took her report seriously. Tick bites seem to trigger this unusual delayed IgE hypersensitivity, but how? The red meat is rich in alpha-gal, and the tick seems to break an already established meat tolerance, causing the immune system to attack what was previously ignored.

One way to hypothesize how the tick (ectoparasite) pulls off this meat allergy is to consider the tick bite as a kind of inadvertent bad vaccine reaction – an unintended consequence of altered immune response. When the tick feeds on the host, alpha-gal leaks from its mouth into the wound. This exposes the victim's immune system to alpha-gal and prompts the immune system to overreact when eating meat. Once sensitized, these patients can no longer tolerate mammal meats such as beef, pork and lamb.

Allergic sensitization to alpha-gal poses a greater risk of arterial plaques, a hallmark of heart disease. The big unanswered question: why is meat allergy on the rise today? Some of the theories include climate change, northward movement of ticks, changes in ticks' microbiome due to pesticides and herbicides, a decline in natural predators, etc.

Our distant ancestors once made alpha-gal as a part of cell membrane components, but modern humans do not have alpha-gal during their evolution to the new modern world. Perhaps a genetic selective advantage may backfire on some susceptible people? Malarial plasmodium parasite – a protozoal parasite – has been the single greatest force shaping the human genome in our evolutionary history, and it is fully coated in alpha-gal. Parasites coated with alpha-gal, tick bites, and development of meat allergies are not accidents, but accidents waiting to happen with the collusion of environmental changes, changes in microbiomes, and the maladaptation of the immune system.

The target of these IgE antibodies may not be the alpha-gal in the meat you have eaten for dinner, but the alpha-gal complex that leaks into circulation from the parasites dwelling in your gut. **A leading explanation holds that we develop more allergies now because our immune systems have become more sensitive to what they encounter,** not because they are exposed to more pollens or allergenic foods than in the past.

I covered food allergy topics previously in my articles, "Parasites and Allergies: Paradise Lost in a Parallel Universe," "Parasites and Allergies-Similarity of Symptoms," and "Food Allergies - Often Overlooked Contributors to Chronic Illness." The only reliable proof we have for the cause and effect of the parasites and allergies relationship is based on clinical observation of the improvement of allergy symptoms with properly-prescribed parasite medications.

Beware how a tick bite can alter your immune response and trigger meat allergy. It is still a mystery. The good news is that, provided you are not bitten by another tick again, sometimes the meat allergy fades on its own. When you get rid of intestinal parasites, restore the microbiome and repair leaky gut, you can handle many mysterious food allergies and the new emerging meat allergy.

Parasites and Mental Illness: Delusions of Parasitosis

For those diagnosed by traditional medicine as having "Delusions of Parasitosis:" read this article. Your condition may not be what others say it is.

Are you one of those people constantly worrying about parasite infestation? You are not alone. There are millions of people suffering from the "delusion" of parasites invading their body, crawling under their skin, nibbling their flesh, and taking away all the nutrients from their body. Typical patients are white women over 40 and well educated with no obvious cognitive impairment or signs of psychiatric disorder. Many people are labeled with a psychiatric condition of "Delusions of Parasitosis," but are they properly diagnosed?

Most of the patients go first to their family physician and then to an array of specialists that could include: 1) an internist specializing in infectious disease, 2) a parasitologist, 3) every known specialist based on their symptoms such as a dermatologist or proctologist or others and 4) eventually seeing psychiatrists.

The diagnosis of "Delusions of Parasitosis" is finally confirmed when all diagnostic tests fail to support the patient's history, condition and complaints. Patients are usually angry and hostile for being given this diagnosis. Psychotherapy is very limited. A psychiatrist may end up resorting to antipsychotic medication to control the patient's "delusions." Dr. Hulda Clark's name is often mentioned for describing this recent phenomenon of diagnostic labeling of "Delusions of Parasitosis."

Before we make any assumption on a final diagnosis of "Delusions of Parasitosis," we need to ask, "Does conventional medicine really use the proper tools to uncover parasitic infestations?" One of their primary, if not sole, tests is a microbiology lab test. How reliable is this test? This test of routine stool evaluation for ova and parasites picks up less than 10% of active infections. There are hundreds of parasites with very complicated life cycles that can exist outside the intestinal tract. Therefore they wouldn't be detected by this test. Many of these parasites can penetrate through skin, lung, nostril and every known organ and tissue in the body.

The World Health Organization (WHO) states that 2 billion people have worms which are rarely seen in the stool exam. I believe those numbers are very conservative. I believe those numbers are limited to worms and nematodes and not inclusive of all parasitic infestations. The WHO estimates that 1.5 billion people worldwide suffer from a neuropsychiatric disorder. Of the 10 leading causes of disability in 1990, four were psychiatric disorders: major depression, manic bipolar depression, schizophrenia and obsessive-compulsive disorders.

The cause of psychiatric disorders and mental illness has been hotly debated and controversial. It has included genetics, nutrition, environmental toxins, drugs, and one's family environment. A minority of physicians and therapists believe there is overwhelming evidence that infectious agents may play a key role in causing mental illness. Dr. E. Fuller Torrey, former professor of psychiatry at the Uniformed Services University in Bethesda, MD wrote a book, "The Invisible Plague: The Rise of Mental Illness from 1750 to the Present." He is a big proponent of linking mental illness with infectious agents as a key cause of mental illness reaching its current epidemic proportions.

Most well-known common infections capable of producing mental illness or its symptoms include syphilis, Lyme disease, pneumonia, urinary tract infections, sepsis, malaria, HIV, Legionnaires Disease, chlamydia, typhoid fever, herpes, tapeworms, giardia, ascariasis, trichinosis, toxoplasmosis, and streptococcal infections. Some of the symptoms are transient after the acute infection, and some are followed by a long protracted disabling sequence of physical and mental breakdown.

Some specific correlations have been observed. Streptococcal infection has been associated with the onset of Obsessive Compulsive Disorder. Toxoplasma gondii has been known to cause delusions, psychosis and auditory hallucinations. Dr. Paul Fink, past president of the American Psychiatric Association, has acknowledged that Lyme disease alone has been known to mimic every known psychiatric diagnosis in the Diagnostic and Statistical Manual of Mental Disorders (DSM). It is interesting to note that many antipsychotic medications have antiviral and antiparasitic activities. Maybe these actions of the medications are the real reason for a reduction in psychotic conditions, at least in some percentage of people.

We are at a crossroads between 21st century conventional medical science and integrative medicine. Many people are suffering from psychiatric problems and receiving anti-psychiatric medications for the wrong reasons and a wrong diagnosis. Perhaps believing that medical science sponsored by pharmaceutical companies is impartial and fair is a delusion in itself. Patients suffer from the delusion of parasitosis. Therapists suffer from the delusion of blind faith on double blind randomized medical trial studies.

Maybe there are two opposing delusions: Delusions of Parasitosis and Delusions of the Merits of Science. Perhaps Hulda Clark was right all along that parasites and all disease known to humans have intimately evolved together. It might be worthwhile to deworm everybody. You could ask your Veterinarian to deworm your cats, dogs, children and you. Or you could take a less radical approach and ask your integrative medical practitioner for parasite remedies for your "Delusions of Parasitosis."

Chapter 8 Fungal Invaders

Fungus is our chief undertaker.

Fungi and molds are additional overlooked stealth invaders that have a dramatic impact on health and disease.

Introduction to Fungi

In a nutshell, a fungus is a symbiont (living in synergy) with plants, animals, or other fungi. However, it can also act as a parasite. A fungus is a eukaryotic organism (which contains a nucleus) that includes unicellular microorganisms such as yeasts and molds, as well as multicellular fungi known as mushrooms. Fungi and early parasites (protozoa) have been evolving over one billion years. "Fungus is among us" as much as parasites are among us. Fungi are genetically more closely related to animals than to plants.

Molds are a bit more complex. A mold is a fungus that grows in the form of multicellular filaments called hyphae. Fungi can be in a single cell as yeast or multiple cells as molds (dimorphic), depending on the conditions in which they grow. Like all fungi, molds derive energy not through photosynthesis but from the organic matter on which they live by recycling the dead or dying organisms – that would be the patient, the host.

Pathogenic fungi produce mycotoxins, toxic metabolites capable of causing disease – and confounding other diseases. They can impact the immune system, kidneys, liver, blood, heart, lymph, and neurological systems, and cause tremors, brain fog and cognitive problems.

Introduction to Mold and Mycotoxin Illnesses

Ritchie Shoemaker, MD's book, *Surviving Mold: Life in the Era of Dangerous Buildings*, provides detailed information on causes, symptoms, diagnosis, and treatment of mold and mycotoxin illnesses, as well as the need for remediation of water-damaged buildings to end external exposure. He frames the impacts of mold and mycotoxins on illnesses in our immune systems, in which we inherit gene variants that make it easier, or harder, to withstand these intruders and mount a hearty defense, or face an unhealthy collapse – what he calls chronic inflammatory response syndrome.

Neil Nathan, MD's book, *Toxic: Heal Your Body from Mold Toxicity, Lyme Disease, Multiple Chemical Sensitivities, and Chronic Environmental Illness*, begins by outlining the concepts of environmental sensitivity and environmental toxicity. He explains their similarities and differences, and how they vary based on our genetics and history of exposures. Impacts on the immune system make it harder to fight off other infections, leading to multiple systems breakdown and the need to "reboot" them for health.

My take is that rebooting our systems includes an energetic component to reset and restore healthy functions in biology as well as in computers, so physicians' plans for effective systems reboots can be guided by Acupuncture Meridian Assessment. Biological dentists play a vital role in systems reboots, as one cannot reboot the body without addressing the teeth, jaw and oral cavity, given its intricate interconnections, interferences and impacts.

Established fungal infections inside the body are a serious health threat. Recent research shows they can damage and induce genetic mutations, causing certain cancers. Aflatoxin b1, the most toxic carcinogen produced by fungi (Aspergillus flavus and Aspergillus parasiticus) that grow on crops such as corn, peanuts, cottonseed, and tree nuts, can cause p53 gene mutations, which are identified in over 50 percent of all human cancers. The p53 gene acts as a tumor suppressor and prevents cells with mutated or damaged DNA from dividing, thereby helping prevent the development of tumors. You can read more in my articles later in this chapter.

Fungal and parasite infections often occur together, and both must be treated with specific medications. In addition, binders such as cholestyramine or charcoal may be used to help remove mycotoxins from the body. Molds are increasingly implicated in environmental illnesses that degrade patients' immune systems and play a role in some cancers and chronic diseases. In the case of exposure to toxic mold – home, school, workplace or other – ongoing exposure must be ended and/or the site thoroughly remediated for recovery to be sustained.

The Dental, Fungal and Parasite Conundrum

What is a conundrum? By definition, it means "a riddle whose answer is or involves a pun" (Merriam-Webster's Dictionary), or "a confusing and difficult problem" (Oxford Dictionary). The definition is vague and not clear to me, but somehow, I find the word "conundrum" fascinating, as well as ambiguous and mysterious. I refer to the process of uncovering three of the most often overlooked, underlying factors fueling cancer and chronic diseases, *"The Dental, Fungal and Parasite Conundrum."*

Why? When listening to chronically ill patients on their first visit – patients who have already seen a long list of specialists and alternative health practitioners – the long, agonizing misadventure of medical histories can be quite confusing, ambiguous and mysterious: a conundrum of life.

As patients share elaborate detailed histories with the latest diagnoses and lab test results, including genetic DNA tests and information on MTHFR methylation pathways, my mind wanders off to the world of the conundrum: a quantum world of what-ifs and a myriad of unknown possibilities...

By the time patients are evaluated by Mayo Clinic or Cleveland Clinic and still have an unknown or mysterious illness (they may give it a fancy idiopathic Latin medical diagnosis), they most likely have some combination of unrecognized dental problems, parasites, and fungal infections producing mycotoxins and their far-reaching effects.

Article: Molds – Enigma of Indoor Pollution

If you are suffering from troubling health problems and your doctor said everything is fine according to lab tests, think mold. Treat the source – and yourself as well.

If you are suffering from headaches, allergies, asthma, fatigue, fibromyalgia, poor memory, persistent cough, muscle weakness, or hypertension, and your doctor said everything is fine according to lab tests, think of environmentally induced illness, especially indoor pollution. Indoor pollution arising within one's home, not outdoor pollution, may be the real reason for chronic illness in susceptible individuals.

Some major sources of indoor contaminants include odors and fumes arising from leaking utility gas or oil pipes for heating furnaces, paint odors, household cleansers and disinfectants, new carpets, bedding and upholstery, and insecticides, pesticides, and fungicides used inside and outside of the home.

Consider the following example of environmentally induced illness. Here are the circumstances: Your house has a history of a leaky roof or basement. You develop shortness of breath, persistent cough or vague chest pain. Your doctor diagnosed you with asthma. You are not responding to asthma medication. You wonder what the cause of your symptoms could be. Consider an allergic reaction to molds. Allergic bronchopulmonary aspergillosis, a mold-induced allergic reaction, can essentially mimic asthma. If this is the case with your condition, it may respond to antifungal drug therapy whereas it did not respond to standard asthma medication.

Stachybotrys fungus, the black mold you might see in your bathroom, in a leaky basement or behind leaky wallpaper, can produce a mycotoxin called trichothecenes. This neurotoxin in a susceptible individual will create a multitude of symptoms. At some point you will say, "My doctor said everything is fine. Then, why do I feel so lousy?" and go through a living hell because of the conditions within your own home.

Is there any hope for environmental illness induced by indoor pollution? First, you have to recognize that the multitude of unexplainable symptoms from which you are suffering might be related to indoor pollution.

Second, you need professional experts to help identify the problems in your home and fix them at the source. If you smell the odor of gas, call the gas company. If you smell moldy odors in your bathroom, you may need to inspect the wall behind the wallpaper. If black or green mold is present, you can hire a professional to clean it up, or remove, remediate and replace it as needed. For people highly sensitive to mold, it is highly recommended to contract with a licensed professional. If you decide to clean it yourself, use a professional grade gas mask to protect your airway and lungs while using a dedicated mold removal product, such as Concrobium. While bleach kills mold, the dead spores it leaves behind can still cause health impacts.

Third, you need proper medical care for your unique exposure to indoor pollution. If you have been exposed to molds and mycotoxins, you may need a trial of antifungal remedies, and use a lab such as Great Plains to check for your level of mycotoxins.

The signs and symptoms of indoor pollution are a big enigma for patients and doctors. If the source of the problem can be identified and corrected, the rewards can be dramatic and enduring.

Article: Fungus, Molds and Mycotoxins: International Mycotoxin Summit in Dallas

From the 2016 International Summit on Mycotoxin Treatments: fungus and molds cause mutations, genetic fusion and fuel cancer. Fungi and mycotoxins can promote cancers by integrating their DNA into human cells, like viruses! Antifungal drugs can help.

Studying fungus (mycology) was not the most exciting subject during my medical school studies. However, problems associated with fungi, molds, and their byproducts, mycotoxins, have been exploding as a hot topic for the last 20 years. I've written many articles on parasites, but fewer articles on fungi and molds.

Fungi are considered a separate kingdom, distinct from both plants and animals. The kingdom of Fungi has been estimated at 1.5 to 5 million species, with about 5 percent of these formally classified. Yeasts are single-celled fungal organisms. The most well-known are brewer's yeast, baker's yeast, and Candida albicans.

Brewer's and baker's yeast are probably the earliest domesticated organisms by mankind for baking breads and brewing beers and wines, going back to Biblical times. C. albicans is an opportunistic pathogen which can cause infections in humans, especially with the introduction of antibiotics and a high-sugar/carbohydrate diet.

These molds reproduce by producing large numbers of small spores which may contain either a single nucleus or multiple nuclei. Mold spores can be asexual (the product of mitosis), sexual (the product of meiosis), or both, and can produce mycotoxins. This information may seem irrelevant to you now, but may be vital information later for unexplainable illnesses in environmentally sensitive patients and physicians caring for them.

The 2016 International Summit on Mycotoxin Treatments was held in Dallas, Texas. The conference covered a broad spectrum of mycotoxin-related illnesses and treatment plans. I went there to refresh my knowledge of mycotoxin-related human illnesses. Among many excellent speakers at the Mycotoxin Treatments Conference, Doug Kaufmann's lecture, "Role of Fungal Mycotoxins in Cancer" was outstanding: a direct, to-the-point, and relevant lecture for why we are getting sick. Highlights include:

The American Cancer Society defines fungal mycotoxins as genotoxic carcinogens. Fungal exposure has been greatly accelerated by sealing our homes, use of heating/air conditioning systems that encourage mold growth, erroneous promotion of grains in the Food Pyramid Charts over the last 70 years, increased alcohol consumption, and the uncontrolled, widespread use of antibiotics in animals and humans.

Mycotoxins can damage and induce **cancer via genetic mutations** at the c-myc oncogene, a master regulator, the N-Ras protein which acts like a switch, and the c-K-Ras oncogene; under certain circumstances, oncogenes have the potential to cause cancer. Fungal spores can survive phagocytosis (being eaten up) by white blood cells by a thick viscous capsule. Paradoxically, white blood cells may protect fungus from other defenses of the host and are instrumental for the spread of cancer/fungal cells, ultimately assisting in metastasis – spreading – to other organs in the body.

The most well-known mycotoxins are aflatoxins, ochratoxins, fumonisins, deoxynivalenol, and zearalenones. These grain mycotoxins will glow green under UV black light. Pathologist Migdalia Arnan, MD describes green granules glowing within human cancer tissues when exposed to UV black light.

Mycotoxins not only cause genetic mutations but also promote genetic fusion, called karyogamy, the final step in the process of fusing together two haploid (half a complete set) DNA of human and fungal cells. **Fungi and mycotoxins** can promote human cancers by **integrating their DNA into human cells like viruses**. The Epstein-Barr virus, papilloma viruses, and hepatitis B and C viruses have been known to promote human cancers by integrating their DNA into human cells.

Research by Blake T. Aftab et al. found that antifungal drugs like itraconazole can stop cancer from metastasizing by inhibiting angiogenesis and slowing tumor growth rate.[27] Scientists at the German Cancer Research Center have discovered that the antifungal drug, griseofulvin, forces cancer cells into death.[28]

*   *   *

Fungal, mold and mycotoxin-related problems can be detected at the allergy/immunology point during evaluation by Acupuncture Meridian Assessment.

Article: Hurricanes, Molds and Death: Don't Mess with Molds, the Undertaker

The CDC urges healthcare providers to "think fungus" when symptoms of infection do not get better with treatment. Given the growing pace of hurricanes and flooding which leave mold and fungus in their wake for years to come, this is timely. It would be great for CDC to add parasites as an awareness campaign!

The U.S. Centers for Disease Control and Prevention (CDC) declared the first Fungal Disease Awareness Week in August 2017 and the second in October 2018, urging healthcare providers and their patients to "think fungus" when symptoms of infection do not get better with treatment. This call to action was timely, as hurricanes are leaving mold and fungus problems in their wake for years to come. Problems associated with fungus, molds, and their byproducts – mycotoxins – have been exploding as a hot topic for the last 20 years. And they are exploding in the United States.

Molds and mycotoxins play an important role in environmental illnesses, as a result of exposure in flooded, damp and leaky homes, schools and workplaces. Patients with unexplained illnesses who do not respond well to treatment may have their immune systems under attack, and may have genetic variants that make them more susceptible to health impacts. Effective treatment requires removal of exposure – and professional testing and remediation of the building – along with prescription antifungals, other remedies, and binders in some cases.

Molds are increasingly implicated in environmental illnesses that degrade patients' immune systems, and fungi are somewhat infamous for contaminating medications. Fungi also play a stealth role in certain cancers. At my 2017 Tenth International Medical Conference, Doug Kaufmann's talk on "The Fungal Etiology of

Cancer" was outstanding. He has written many books, including *The Germ That Causes Cancer*. Other speakers on this topic included Lee Cowden, MD, and John Trowbridge, MD, author of the pathbreaking book, *The Yeast Syndrome*. CDs or DVDs of the conference talks are at www.Aurora Recording.com.

Fungal mycotoxins are genotoxic, mutagenic, immunosuppressive, tremorgenic, neurotoxic, nephrotoxic, hepatotoxic, hemotoxic, cardiotoxic, lymphotoxic, and dermatotoxic. Aflatoxin b1 is the most hepatotoxic carcinogen, and the most potent natural carcinogen known, and is commonly found in foods such as peanuts and grains.

Fungal infections can mimic many cancers, including lung cancer and skin cancer. The mycotoxin aflatoxin b1 is known to cause p53 gene mutations. The p53 gene codes for a protein that regulates the cell cycle and is known to protect against cancer proliferation. The damage to p53 allows cells with damaged DNA to proliferate. The p53 mutation is identified in over 50 percent of all human cancers.

Fungi and mycotoxins can promote human cancers by integrating their DNA into human cells like viruses. The Epstein-Barr virus, papilloma viruses, and hepatitis B and C viruses are known to promote human cancers by integrating their DNA into human cells.

Parasites and fungus evolve and often coexist. When using antiparasitic and antifungal medications, I have observed stabilization of tumor growth and at times, spontaneous remission, which I call "accidental cure."

I cannot wait for the CDC to declare the first "Parasite Disease Awareness Month" which consists of "Virus, Bacteria, Fungus, and Mycobacteria Awareness Week!" Parasites are the top of the food chain, and fungus is our chief undertaker.

Part 4
Contesting Cancer, Lyme and Mystery Diseases

Chapter 9 Cancer: What Are We Missing?

We can treat cancer, not based on genetic mutations,
but based on a common global mitochondrial
property that is characteristic of cancer stem cells.

Cancer is the second leading cause of death in America: a close second after heart disease, it accounts for nearly 25% of the total. Currently, nearly 40% of men and 38% of women develop cancer during their lifetime.[29] The term "cancer" provokes anxiety and fear of a slow, painful inevitable death for millions of people every year. Images of a disfigured body, drawn-out chemotherapy, radiation and financial distress create even more apprehension for cancer patients and their families.

The War on Cancer has been a rocky road, with some significant advances, yet progress not as far or as fast as hoped. The number of cancer survivors in the U.S. has increased from 3 million in 1971 to 15.5 million in 2015.[30] However, this number can be misleading. Death rates are falling due to early detection leading to a rise in the numbers diagnosed and treated, yet incidence rates and the number of deaths continue to rise for some cancers.[31] Cancer incidence also varies by gender and race.[32][33] About 1.7 million new cancer cases were projected to be diagnosed in 2018, and an estimated 609,640 people died of cancer in 2018.[34]

We are losing the official War on Cancer, yet paint a promising picture of progress. Pharma companies fund patient organizations who lobby for funding for cures, which can be costly, brutal and tough to endure. Many researchers are looking at the genetics of tumors, yet fewer are looking hard at what triggers them.

During the years I have been searching for underlying causes of cancer, my aunt died with lymphoma and my wife's aunt died with lung cancer. They did not die from their cancers. They died while going through chemotherapy. How can I be sure?

As a physician, I have witnessed hundreds of similar cases of relatively stable cancer patients dying soon after or during the course of their surgery, chemotherapy and radiation therapies. Yet, there is a silence among physicians because we feel powerless to help our patients. Is there any other way to help those with cancer? I began to look for and investigate other approaches.

Building on the Foundation in My First Book

After retiring from the U.S. Army Reserves, I started working on my first book, *Accidental Cure: Extraordinary Medicine for Extraordinary Patients,* describing my experiences with a U.S. Army medical operation near Oruro, Bolivia. With extensive use of parasite medications given to native Bolivian Indians, many reported spontaneous healing of other conditions.

I began using the same parasite medications on my patients here in the United States, and I witnessed spontaneous healings from many incurable medical conditions, including some cancers. I also found that detecting and having patients remove hidden dental infections can result in spontaneous healing from certain cancers, as well as from a range of autoimmune and neurological diseases.

Without proof or evidence, such as a detected parasite in a standard stool test, I decided to call these healing phenomena – after one or more rounds of antiparasitic and antifungal medications and/or addressing a hidden dental infection – an "accidental cure."

Unlike the War on Cancer – which many critics have said has been stymied or lost – my battle plans are based on combining U.S.

Army doctrine for military operations and a biocybernetic/energy medicine program. They integrate the best of conventional and integrative medicine, traditional Chinese medicine and acupuncture, and German biological medicine to counter known and unknown asymmetric threats to health.

War on Cancer

The "War on Cancer" effectively began with Congress enacting and President Richard Nixon signing the National Cancer Act of 1971, though it was not described as a "war" in the legislation itself. The Act strengthened and provided funding to the National Cancer Institute. For a narrative history of the War on Cancer, see Siddhartha Mukherjee's *The Emperor of All Maladies*, made into a PBS documentary by Ken Burns.

In 2003, Andrew von Eschenbach, then director of the National Cancer Institute, challenged the United States "to eliminate suffering and death due to cancer by 2015."[35] We have not met this goal. At the same time, there is increasing knowledge of some of the causes of some cancers and actions to lower risk. The American Cancer Society cites cancers caused by tobacco use and heavy alcohol consumption, obesity, physical inactivity, and poor nutrition; infectious agents such as human papillomavirus (HPV), hepatitis B and C viruses, HIV, Helicobacter pylori (H. pylori); and skin cancers caused by excessive sun exposure. It notes the importance of screening and early detection.

Marketing of Hope and Fear

There has been a successful marketing of both hope and fear by the medical-pharmaceutical industry. Patient groups receive funding and in turn lobby for more research. High-profile medical institutions have convinced the public that cancer is far too complex, with mysterious oncogene dysregulations, for the average person to understand and primary care physicians to treat.

As a result, only cancer specialists in hospitals are qualified to take care of cancer patients, with support and enforcement by government agencies such as the Department of Health and Human Services (HHS), Centers for Disease Control and Prevention (CDC), Food and Drug Administration (FDA), and National Institutes of Health (NIH).

What is Cancer?

In a nutshell, cancer is the uncontrolled growth of cells. According to the NIH's National Cancer Institute (NCI), cancer is a term for "diseases in which abnormal cells divide without control and can invade nearby tissues. Cancer cells can also spread to other parts of the body through the blood and lymph systems."[36]

There are several main types of cancer.

- Carcinoma, the most common form, begins in epithelial cells, in skin or in tissues that line or cover internal organs.
- Sarcoma begins in bone, cartilage, fat, muscle, blood vessels, or other connective or supportive tissue.
- Leukemia starts in blood-forming tissue, such as bone marrow, and causes large numbers of abnormal blood cells to be produced and enter the blood.
- Lymphoma and multiple myeloma begin in the cells of the immune system.
- Central nervous system cancers begin in the tissues of the brain and spinal cord.

More basics:

Cancer tumors are malignant, and can spread into or invade nearby tissues. As tumors grow, some cancer cells can break off and travel to distant places in the body through the blood or lymph system and form new tumors far from the original site, in a process called **metastasis**. In contrast, benign tumors are generally not harmful.

Cancer cells are less specialized than normal cells. While normal cells mature into very distinct cell types with specific functions, cancer cells do not. This is one reason that cancer cells continue to divide without stopping.

Cancer cells ignore signals that normally tell cells to stop dividing, or to begin a process of programmed cell death – **apoptosis** – which the body uses to rid it of unneeded cells.

Cancer cells may be able to influence normal cells, molecules, and blood vessels that surround and feed a tumor. For instance, cancer cells can induce nearby normal cells to form blood vessels, called **angiogenesis**, that supply tumors with oxygen and nutrients, which they need to grow. The blood vessels also remove waste products from tumors.

Cancer cells are also often able to evade the immune system. Although the immune system normally removes damaged or abnormal cells from the body, some cancer cells are able to "hide" from the immune system.

Cancer tumors can also use the immune system to stay alive and grow. For example, with the help of certain immune system cells that normally prevent a runaway immune response, cancer cells can actually keep the immune system from killing cancer cells.[37]

Tricky, isn't it? What an asymmetric threat we face in cancer!

Cancer Risk Factors and Causes

According to the National Cancer Institute (NCI), risk factors and causes of cancer include:

- Age
- Alcohol
- Cancer-Causing Substances
- Chronic Inflammation
- Diet
- Hormones
- Immunosuppression
- Infectious Agents
- Obesity
- Radiation
- Sunlight
- Tobacco

Some of these are within your control, but many others are not.

Cancer-causing substances include not only well-known toxins like cigarette smoke and asbestos, but also aflatoxins – mycotoxins produced by fungi, Aspergillus flavus and Aspergillus parasiticus, found on agricultural crops such as corn, peanuts, cottonseed, and tree nuts. Aflatoxins are associated with liver cancer.[38]

Chronic inflammation may be caused by infections that don't go away, abnormal immune reactions to normal tissues, or conditions such as obesity. Over time, chronic inflammation can cause DNA damage and lead to cancer. For example, people with chronic inflammatory bowel diseases, such as ulcerative colitis and Crohn's disease, have an increased risk of colon cancer. Dental infections are the most commonly overlooked sources of inflammation by oncologists.[39]

Certain **infectious agents**, including viruses, bacteria, fungi and parasites can cause cancer or increase the risk that cancer will form. Some viruses can disrupt signaling that normally keeps cell growth and proliferation in check. Some infections weaken the immune system, making the body less able to fight off other cancer-causing infections. Some viruses, bacteria, fungi, and parasites cause chronic inflammation, which may lead to cancer.

- Epstein-Barr Virus (EBV) – virus: lymphoma, nose and throat cancer
- Hepatitis B Virus and Hepatitis C Virus (HBV and HCV) – virus: liver cancer
- Human Immunodeficiency Virus (HIV) – virus: weakens immunity, raises risk of cancer
- Human Papillomaviruses (HPVs) – virus: cervical cancer
- Human T-Cell Leukemia/Lymphoma Virus Type 1 (HTLV-1) – virus: non-Hodgkin's lymphoma
- Kaposi Sarcoma-Associated Herpesvirus (KSHV) – virus: Kaposi sarcoma
- Merkel Cell polyomavirus (MCPyV) – virus: Merkle Cell skin cancer
- Helicobacter pylori (H. pylori) – bacteria: stomach cancer, gastric lymphoma, ulcers
- Opisthorchis viverrini – parasitic flatworm (fluke): bile duct cancer
- Schistosoma haematobium – parasitic flatworm (fluke): bladder cancer[40]

Early efforts to eradicate and treat cancers focused on surgery, chemotherapy and radiation, ways to remove and kill fast-growing tumor cells. Cut it out, carpet bomb it, scorch the earth around it, and deprive it of fuel: surgery, chemotherapy, radiation, and tamoxifen-type anti-estrogens seek to prevent and arrest cancer cells' spread and future growth. Treatments have expanded to include hormone therapy, immune therapy, and targeted therapy (drugs that interfere specifically with cancer cell growth).

The Human Genome Project and the Precision Medicine Initiative led to targeting of cancer treatments by tumor gene type. The Cancer Moonshot further expands the search for treatments to immunotherapy, super-charging the body's own immune system to fight cancers. Yet limits, risks (including death) and side effects, while delivering hope and results for some patients, continue to challenge and disappoint those who do not respond well, along with families, physicians and researchers. What are we missing?

New Research and Treatment Strategies

Hidden problems that can trigger the development of cancers include dental infections, fungi, and parasites. This was a major theme at my 10th International Integrative Medicine Conference, *Curing the Incurables: Fungal Parasites Dental Conundrum.*

Researcher Doug Kaufmann gave a presentation, "The Fungal Etiology of Cancer." In his journey from fungal-infected Vietnam War veteran to medical researcher, Kaufmann learned about fungi's role in a wide range of human health problems: behavioral, diabetes, gut, heart problems, and cancers. He believes cancer is overdiagnosed; many are fungal infections and improve with antifungal therapy. He described his Kaufmann Cancer Hypothesis: fungal and human DNA merge to form cancer cells. Kaufmann's work to promote antifungal, anticancer diets is attracting greater attention in the medical community.

Research led by Rossitza Lazova of Yale School of Medicine and others shows that metastasis occur when white blood cells – leukocytes – and cancer cells fuse and form a genetic hybrid.[41]

Kaufmann outlined his protocols for using antifungals and diet to help prevent and treat certain cancers and chronic inflammatory diseases, which are on his website, www.knowthecause.com.

Christine Salter, MD, DC, of the Center for Vibrant Health and Wellness in St. Louis, presented case studies of fungal problems linked to chronic diseases. She said it is time to get the elephant off the foot, because interleukin 12 (IL-12), an immune system cytokine-signaling molecule which plays an important role in activating natural killer cells and inhibiting angiogenesis (new blood vessel formation), is inhibited by mycotoxins. After learning about fungal connections to cancer, she began treating lymph and metastatic cancer patients with antifungal medications and diet. If not successful in resolving the cancer, she refers to oncology.

Antonio Jimenez, MD, ND, CNC, and Chief Medical Officer of Hope4Cancer Institute in Mexico, introduced *The Pathogenic Sphere of Cancer*. He surveyed research on cancer microbes with characteristics similar to fungi, cell-wall-deficient forms of bacteria, stealth pathogens, parasites, and viruses such as human cytomegalovirus (HCMV). HCMV is a herpes virus which is common, but can be dangerous to those with weakened immune systems. In cancer, HCMV could favor the progression and spread of the tumor, a concept called "oncomodulation."

Jimenez said that eliminating pathogens is needed for the 15-20 percent of cancers that are linked to infections, produce toxins, encourage loss of cellular control, and evade the immune system. Why? Pathogens release cancer-causing, mutagenic cytokine-signaling molecules. Reviewing a variety of treatment strategies, we need a multimodal approach to restore the body's terrain.

Search for Underlying Causes of Cancer

Years ago, I wrote an article, "Nutritional Therapies for Cancer," to provide my patients with ways and means to fight cancer with a broader toolkit, including nutrition and detoxification. It gave tips on how to look for unsuspected hidden problems that might be overlooked and serve as additional underlying causes of cancers that trigger and fuel them to develop, spread and grow.

What have we learned that conventional oncologists overlook?

First, most researchers now agree that while some people have a genetic predisposition to certain cancers, there is typically a trigger or series of triggering events involved. The product of both nature and nurture, cancer is the result of **epigenetic changes** – changes in how genes are expressed – but not the gene type itself.

The evidence linking epigenetic processes with cancer is becoming "extremely compelling," says Peter Jones, director of the University of Southern California's Norris Comprehensive Cancer Center.[42] Toshikazu Ushijima, of Japan's National Cancer Center Research Institute, says epigenetic mechanisms are one of the five most important considerations in the cancer field, and they account for one-third to one-half of known genetic alterations.

Second, cancer is primarily a **metabolic disease**. In addition to genetics, environmental triggers, inflammation and infections, cancer also has metabolic factors which fuel its growth. As you will read in the articles at the end of this chapter:

All forms of infectious microbes, including viruses, bacteria, and parasites, can create an inflammatory immune response which can, under toxic environmental conditions, cause cancer cells to grow.

Bone marrow-derived stem cells have "cancer-like properties." These include the capacity for unlimited growth, ability to avoid programmed cell death signals, and capacity to develop into many tissue types. To transform into cancer, the trigger can be chronic inflammation from a pre-existing bacterial infection, such as Helicobacter pylori (causes ulcers). Damage to the stomach lining also plays a role.

Cancer cells rely on glucose (sugar) as the predominant source of energy for survival. This is referred to as the Warburg effect. Dr. Otto Warburg proved that glycolysis fermentation is the hallmark of cancer regardless of tissue origin. Glycolysis is the first stop in the breakdown of glucose to extract energy for cellular metabolism.

According to Thomas Seyfried, PhD, most cancer, regardless of cell or tissue origin, is a disease of respiratory insufficiency coupled with compensatory glycolysis fermentation. **Cancer cells need glucose and glutamine. Restricting** them per a low-sugar, low-carb, and ketogenic-type diet can help.

Ivermectin may be able to clear up some cancers. At higher doses, it can inactivate protein kinase PAK1, block growth of ovarian cancer and neurofibromatosis type 2 (NF2) tumor cells, and help chemotherapy kill leukemia cells.

Recent research has found that antibiotics that target mitochondria can effectively eradicate cancer stem cells across multiple tumor types: treating cancer like an infectious disease. There is an **Achilles' heel** in cancer stem cells' mitochondria. Because mitochondria evolved from bacteria that were originally engulfed by early eukaryotic-protozoa cells over one billion years ago (the endosymbiotic theory of mitochondrial evolution), **cancer**

mitochondria are more susceptible to those classes of mitochondria-targeted antibiotics.

In essence, we can treat cancer, not based on genetic mutations, but based on a common global mitochondrial property that is characteristic of cancer stem cells. This applies to many cancer types. Importantly, azithromycin, tigecycline, and doxycycline are known to cross the blood-brain barrier, making the treatment of brain cancer with these antibiotics potentially feasible.

Insulin Potentiation Therapy (IPT)

In terms of treatment strategies, Insulin Potentiation Therapy (IPT) is another promising approach. Targeted low-dose therapies, accompanied by insulin to starve cancer cells via hypoglycemia, provide a tool to combat cancer. During the episode of hypoglycemia, the physician infuses small amounts of specific medications for that particular medical condition. The dose of the medication can be reduced to 10% of the regular dose.

Cancer cells absorb an IPT sugar-chemotherapy agent solution before it gets to normal cells. Normal cells are minimally affected by low-dose chemotherapy. IPT is equivalent to a **Trojan horse**, bringing the soldiers (remedies) to only the enemy's well-protected cancer cells. Integrative oncologists can administer lower doses of chemotherapy via IPT, minimizing the impact on healthy cells, and minimizing side effects.

I use IPT with a wide range of medications, such as antiparasitics, antifungals, antibiotics, antivirals, and immune boosting nutrients, to target their uptake by cancer cells. I am not an oncologist and do not treat cancer with chemotherapy. I leave that to the oncologists.

Key to Survival: Eliminate Hidden Enemies and Rebuild Healthy Terrain

There have been significant advances in integrative cancer care, which are described further in the articles at the end of this chapter. There are many excellent books on integrative and complementary cancer therapy, and my goal is not to reiterate them. Instead, I look at cancer and cancer management from the perspective of conducting a successful military campaign and tactical operation. This is another way to explain the century-old problem of cancer.

I am a general internist, not an oncologist; I specialize in taking care of chronically sick patients, including cancer patients. I have seen too much unnecessary suffering due to the current standard of cancer care in the United States and around the world. I have learned from my experiences as a physician, as a regional medical director for an HMO, and as a U.S. Army Reserve medical doctor, and I want to share what I have learned. My focus is to isolate asymmetric threats, systematically eliminate hidden enemies in the war against cancer, and rebuild the biological terrain and conditions that support health.

In my own practice, I have treated numerous patients where the cause of a tumor turned out to be parasites, fungi and/or dental problems, and many others where antiparasitic and antifungal medications have been part of my treatment plan, along with a supportive diet and addressing other burdens on the immune system such as heavy metals, toxins and dental infections.

When our physical body is fed a faulty diet, including processed and genetically-altered food, lives in toxic environments, lives with chronic infections, and when we are under constant attack with fear and toxic emotions, our body starts to degenerate. It may manifest as diabetes, heart problems, autoimmune disease, arthritis, or tumors as our bodies become more acidic and toxic. Is it possible to reverse the process of cancerous conditions? It takes more than antibiotics or antiparasitics to treat cancer. We need to treat the whole body on physical, emotional, and spiritual levels.

It is worthwhile to start using natural and prescribed antibiotics, antifungal, and antiparasitic medications as a means to reduce the total burden of infections as a part of cancer management programs by primary care physicians. It may have a secondary benefit of targeting the mitochondria of cancer stem cells. Recent research gives us a glimpse of hope and the possibility of a cure for cancer.

Battle Plan: Joe, Cancer of the Left Leg and Spine

Here is my battle plan for Joe, who came to see me wheelchair-bound with advanced cancer of his left upper leg that spread to his spine. He progressed with therapies and had remission, but did not complete dental work. Fighting cancer is a lifetime commitment.

Chief Complaint

In November 2009, Joe, a 58-year-old man in a wheelchair, came to see me with advanced cancer of his left upper leg that metastasized to his spine. In August 2009, Joe's initial symptoms were left leg pain and low back pain. He also felt a mass in his left thigh. A biopsy of the bone showed moderate to poorly differentiated non-small cell carcinoma of unknown origin. A CT scan of the abdomen and pelvis showed an 11.3 centimeter by 4.3 centimeter mass, multilocular solid and cystic mass to the proximal femur (thigh bone), osseous pattern, lytic, consistent with advanced disease with subcutaneous edema (swelling).

Joe had a positron emission tomography (PET) scan which showed metastases to the lumber spine L-4 and ninth thoracic vertebra T9 bones. The left femur in his upper leg would soon fracture, and a surgeon placed a pin in it for stabilization. Chemotherapy was started but soon stopped because of severe ulceration over his whole body. He was sent home under hospice care. He also complained of night sweats and leg/scrotal swelling and pain.

Physical Exam

At the time of his physical exam in my office, Joe was in a wheelchair and taking pain medication but still in significant distress from the pain in his leg and low back. Acupuncture Meridian Assessment indicated 23 out of 40 main meridians were out of balance, as illustrated in Figure 11. His dominant problems were from the large intestine, liver, stomach and gallbladder meridians, and dental meridian. I consider AMA, a biocybernetic/energetic evaluation, to be a part of my physical exam.

Figure 11. Cancer of Left Leg – Initial AMA Evaluation
Cancer of Left Leg Metastasized to Spine: Nov. 2009
(23 Meridians Out of Balance)

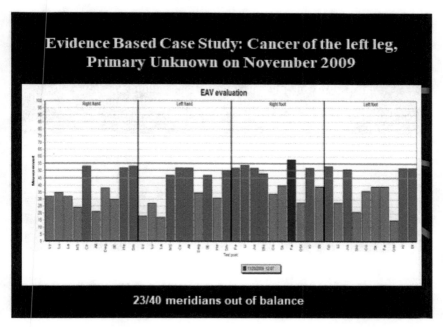

Initial Treatment

Based the information from the Acupuncture Meridian Assessment (AMA), Joe was started on ivermectin 12 mg 4x/day for 10 days, followed by levamisole 50 mg 4x/day for 10 days with instructions to repeat the cycle a few weeks later (levamisole is no longer available due to safety concerns, but niclosamide shows promise).

About six weeks later, on January 3, 2010, after taking the parasite medications, Joe noticed a gradual decrease in swelling of the left thigh, his pain had gradually dissipated, he lost 20 pounds of fluids and mass and was able to walk to the clinic without using the wheelchair. Further AMA testing revealed three of his dental and allergy meridians were out of balance. See Figure 12.

Figure 12. Cancer of Left Leg – Jan. 2010 AMA Results
Cancer of Left Leg Metastasized to Spine:
Dental & Allergy Meridians Out of Balance

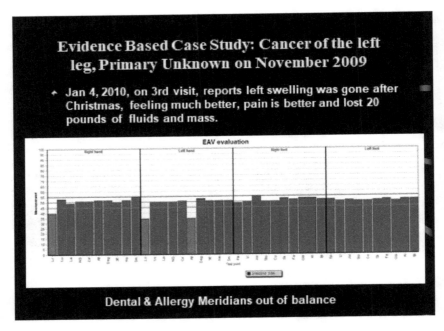

Lab Tests

Additional lab testing revealed his erythrocyte sedimentation rate (ESR or sed rate) test was high at 51. His DMPS heavy metal provocation test revealed very high levels of lead, mercury, tungsten and platinum (from chemotherapy). See Figure 13.

Figure 13. Cancer of Left Leg - Heavy Metals Test
Cancer of Left Leg Metastasized to Spine

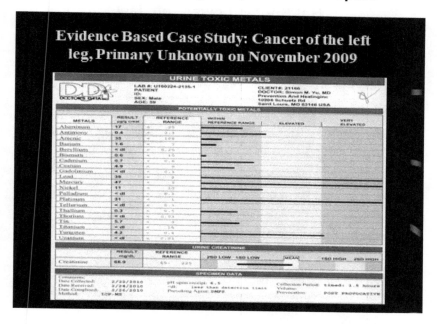

The test results indicate very elevated levels of lead, mercury, platinum and tungsten, and elevated levels of antimony and nickel.

Dental Problems

Far infrared thermal imaging also showed possible dental problems in the left lower quadrant of his mouth. See Figure 14.

Figure 14. Cancer of Left Leg - Head Thermograph
Cancer of Left Leg Metastasized to Spine
Hot Spot in Lower Left Jaw

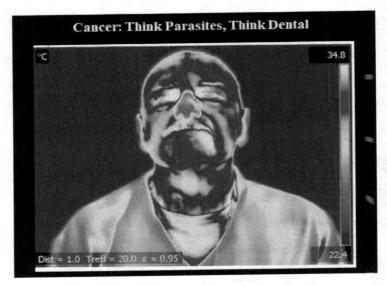

Recommendations

In May 2010, during a visit to see his orthopedic surgeon for the follow-up, Joe was told the x-ray of the left femur revealed the tumor mass was gone and there was no sign of cancer, with a conclusion that there was complete healing.

I instructed Joe to continue oral and IV nutritional therapy, chelation therapy and to complete the dental work to prevent the cancer from coming back. However, he did not come to see me for an entire year, and came back when he was experiencing pain in his right arm.

In March 2011, Joe came back with a new mass on his right arm, indicating metastasis. AMA testing showed three meridians out of balance. See Figure 15.

Figure 15. Cancer of Left Leg - Mar. 2011 AMA Results
Cancer of Left Leg Metastasized to Right Arm
Three Meridians Out of Balance

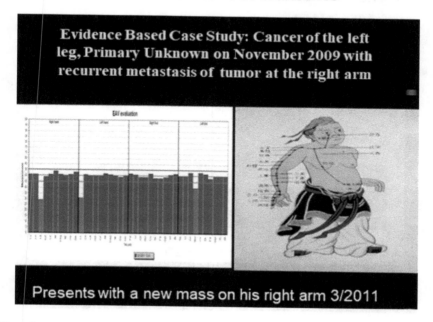

Evidence Based Case Study: Cancer of the left leg, Primary Unknown on November 2009 with recurrent metastasis of tumor at the right arm

Presents with a new mass on his right arm 3/2011

Further Treatment

After additional rounds of parasite medications, his meridians were again in balance. See Figure 16.

Figure 16. Cancer of Left Leg - June 2011 AMA Results
Cancer of Left Leg Metastasized to Right Arm
Meridians in Balance after Parasite Medications

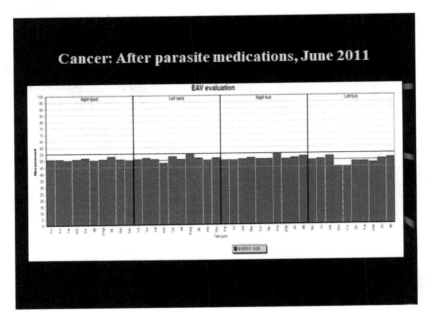

However, Joe did not continue the therapies. When I asked him why, he said he was paying over $2,000/month to keep his medical insurance out of fear, but could not afford to come to see me. He was willing to pay top dollar, which bought him medical care for the chemotherapy. Before I could treat him again, his cancer spread rapidly, he was unable to come to see me for treatment, and Joe died shortly afterwards.

Too often, I see similar cases: a tumor disappears or cancer is stabilized, and a patient stops coming back to continue therapy, most likely for financial reasons and a sense of false security that they have the beaten cancer. In my opinion, once you have cancer, you are required to make a lifetime commitment to battle the cancer.

Battle Plan: Cheryl with Multiple Myeloma

This describes the battle plan for my patient, Cheryl, whose story you read in Chapter 1, The Journey and Quest for Health. Her battle plan includes multiple parasite treatments, dental work and oral surgery, heavy metals chelation, nutritional IV supplements, and ongoing Insulin Potentiation Therapy (IPT). She is doing well.

Cheryl, a 46-year-old woman came to see me with a history of a lump in her neck for one year. Her ENT specialist diagnosed her with plasmacytoma (tumor) of the nasopharynx (between the nasal area and soft palate above the oral cavity), and with multiple myeloma. She was treated with 20 rounds of radiation. However, she was still positive on a PET scan with metastases to multiple bones, biopsy positive for persistent cancer, and an increase in pain. Her physical exam was normal. Acupuncture Meridian Assessment indicated 20 of 40 meridians were out of balance in her initial evaluation. See top half of Figure 17.

Figure 17. Multiple Myeloma - AMA Evaluation Results (20 Meridians Out of Balance Pre-treatment, 3 Out of Balance after Parasite Medications)

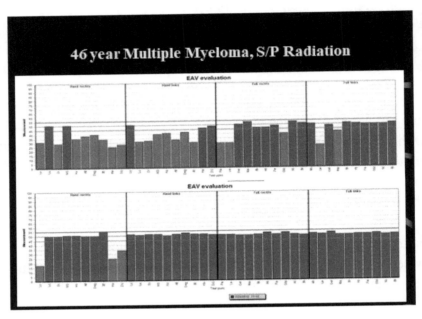

Initial Treatments

Treatment included ivermectin, pyrantel pamoate, praziquantel, artemisinin plus IV vitamin C, IV ozone, UV therapy and dental referral for a biological oral surgeon and holistic oncologist.

Following treatment, three of her meridians were out of balance – primarily dental and allergy/immunology points. See bottom of half of Figure 17.

Dental Problems

A panoramic x-ray gave further evidence of dental problems in her upper left (circled), lower left and right quadrants. See Figure 18.

Figure 18. Multiple Myeloma - Panoramic Dental X-Ray
Woman with Multiple Myeloma
Dental Problems at Upper Left, and Lower Left & Right

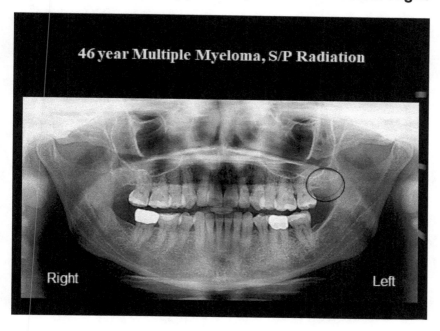

The upper circled area is infected; images reverse left and right.

Heavy Metals

A urine toxic metals test indicated high levels of lead, mercury and thallium. See Figure 19. Cheryl did a program of IV chelation.

Figure 19. Multiple Myeloma - Heavy Metals Test
Woman with Multiple Myeloma
High Levels of Lead, Mercury and Thallium

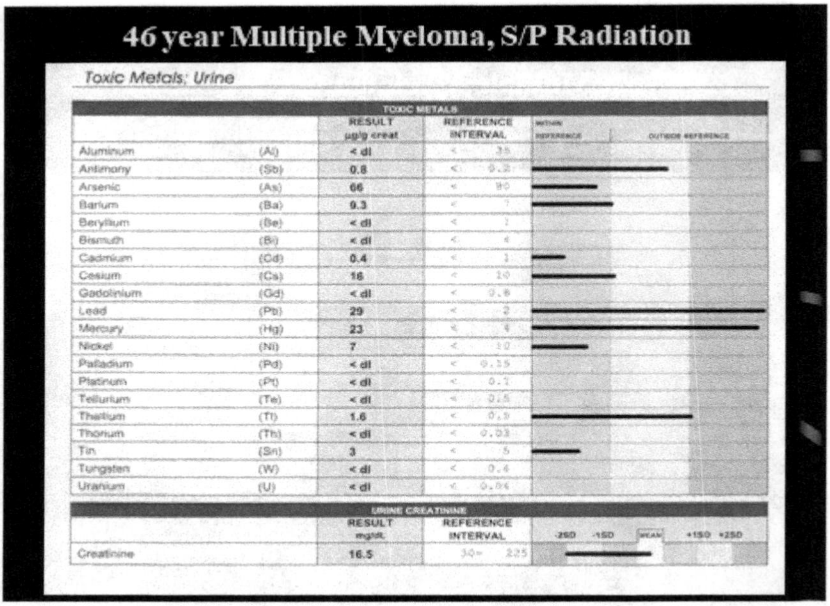

46 year Multiple Myeloma, S/P Radiation

Toxic Metals; Urine

TOXIC METALS		RESULT µg/g creat	REFERENCE INTERVAL	WITHIN REFERENCE / OUTSIDE REFERENCE
Aluminum	(Al)	< dl	< 35	
Antimony	(Sb)	0.8	< 0.2	
Arsenic	(As)	66	< 80	
Barium	(Ba)	9.3	< 7	
Beryllium	(Be)	< dl	< 1	
Bismuth	(Bi)	< dl	< 4	
Cadmium	(Cd)	0.4	< 1	
Cesium	(Cs)	16	< 10	
Gadolinium	(Gd)	< dl	< 0.8	
Lead	(Pb)	29	< 2	
Mercury	(Hg)	23	< 4	
Nickel	(Ni)	7	< 10	
Palladium	(Pd)	< dl	< 0.15	
Platinum	(Pt)	< dl	< 0.1	
Tellurium	(Te)	< dl	< 0.5	
Thallium	(Tl)	1.6	< 0.5	
Thorium	(Th)	< dl	< 0.03	
Tin	(Sn)	3	< 5	
Tungsten	(W)	< dl	< 0.4	
Uranium	(U)	< dl	< 0.04	

URINE CREATININE	RESULT mg/dL	REFERENCE INTERVAL	-2SD -1SD MEAN +1SD +2SD
Creatinine	16.5	30– 225	

Food Antibody Test

Her IgG Food Antibody Assessment showed high reactivity to peanuts and soy. Peanuts are a source of aflatoxins, carcinogens which are produced by certain molds. Soy allergies and sensitivities may be exacerbated by the presence of GMOs and glyphosate. Globally, glyphosate-tolerant soy is the top genetically modified crop plant, representing 75% of total soy production in 2011. See Figure 20.

Figure 20. Multiple Myeloma - Food Antibody Test
Woman with Multiple Myeloma
Food Sensitivity to Peanuts and Soy

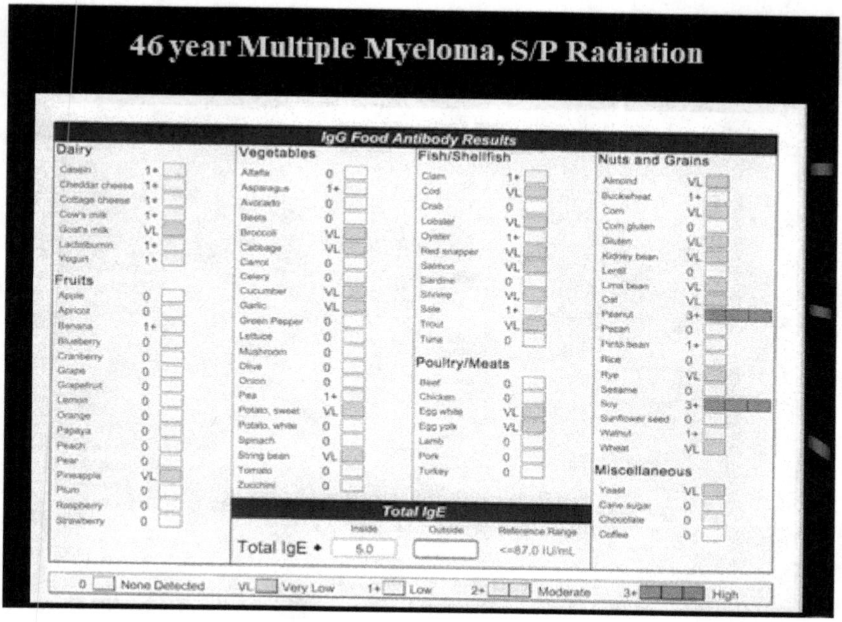

46 year Multiple Myeloma, S/P Radiation

IgG Food Antibody Results

Dairy		Vegetables		Fish/Shellfish		Nuts and Grains	
Casein	1+	Alfalfa	0	Clam	1+	Almond	VL
Cheddar cheese	1+	Asparagus	1+	Cod	VL	Buckwheat	1+
Cottage cheese	1+	Avocado	0	Crab	0	Corn	VL
Cow's milk	1+	Beets	0	Lobster	VL	Corn gluten	0
Goat's milk	VL	Broccoli	VL	Oyster	1+	Gluten	VL
Lactalbumin	1+	Cabbage	VL	Red snapper	VL	Kidney bean	VL
Yogurt	1+	Carrot	0	Salmon	VL	Lentil	0
Fruits		Celery	0	Sardine	0	Lima bean	VL
Apple	0	Cucumber	VL	Shrimp	VL	Oat	VL
Apricot	0	Garlic	VL	Sole	1+	Peanut	3+
Banana	1+	Green Pepper	0	Trout	VL	Pecan	0
Blueberry	0	Lettuce	0	Tuna	0	Pinto bean	1+
Cranberry	0	Mushroom	0	**Poultry/Meats**		Rice	0
Grape	0	Olive	0	Beef	0	Rye	VL
Grapefruit	0	Onion	0	Chicken	0	Sesame	0
Lemon	0	Pea	1+	Egg white	VL	Soy	3+
Orange	0	Potato, sweet	VL	Egg yolk	VL	Sunflower seed	0
Papaya	0	Potato, white	0	Lamb	0	Walnut	1+
Peach	0	Spinach	0	Pork	0	Wheat	VL
Pear	0	String bean	VL	Turkey	0	**Miscellaneous**	
Pineapple	VL	Tomato	0			Yeast	VL
Plum	0	Zucchini	0			Cane sugar	0
Raspberry	0					Chocolate	0
Strawberry	0					Coffee	0

Total IgE

	Inside	Outside	Reference Range
Total IgE ✦	5.0		<=87.0 IU/mL

0 None Detected	VL Very Low	1+ Low	2+ Moderate	3+ High

Insulin Potentiation Therapy Results: Free Kappa Light Chain

Cheryl was treated with multiple rounds of insulin potentiation therapy (IPT). IPT is a promising way to deliver medications using lower dosages and enhance their effectiveness, as cancer cells absorb the agent before it gets to normal cells; see my article, "Insulin Potentiation Therapy," later in this chapter. I gave her antiviral, antifungal, antibacterial and antiparasitic medications via IPT to strengthen her immune system. Her free kappa light chain readings fell from 3,260 to 67 over 16 months. See Figure 21. She continues her treatments, which will be ongoing, and is enjoying her children and family.

Figure 21. Multiple Myeloma - Free Kappa Light Chain
Woman with Multiple Myeloma on Insulin Potentiation Therapy

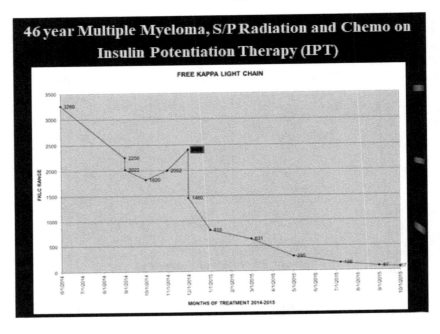

Da's Remarkable Life and Cancer Recovery: Truth, Intuition and God's Will

Here is Da's remarkable story of his life and recent battle with cancer, and help and support from his wife, Sunny, a physician.

I grew up in a poor peasant family in rural China. As a child, I was plagued with belly worms, and they burned coal brick for heat when they ran out of fuel. One day my father, a village acupuncturist, treated the daughter of a Christian Baptist who had a stroke; he didn't ask for money. Her twin sister asked, "What can I do for you?" He said, "Maybe you can teach my son English."

So, I learned English, went to Beijing University, and then to a Christian college in Lincoln, Nebraska. I earned a law degree at Columbia in New York City and worked on Wall Street. Through church, I met my future wife, Sunny, who became a doctor at Loma Linda medical school, and we started a family.

I began writing a book to tell my first-born daughter where I came from. Sunny edited it. I joined a writing group at Barnes and Noble, and they began to read my chapters. One of the group members was an insider who suggested I send it to four agents. One sent it out to nine publishers. By the end of the weekend, all of them vied for it. Random House paid me $500,000. I went on to write eight books.

When Sunny, a conventionally trained physician, developed back pain in 2016, I had convinced her to try acupuncture. She began a journey to learn about integrative approaches to health and medicine. In the fall of 2017, she attended Dr. Yu's "Curing the Incurables" Conference to learn more about dental problems. Shortly before this, I developed neuropathy. Within 2-3 weeks, my left leg became numb.

The week after Sunny returned from the conference, I was diagnosed with brain cancer. Tests revealed I had a 4 cm tumor in my lung, which had metastasized to my brain. Lung cancer is a silent killer. If it had not metastasized, I would not have had a sign. My journey began.

Testing revealed I had non-small cell lung cancer with an epithelial growth factor (EGFR) mutation that could respond to the targeted immunotherapy drug afatinib. I began that treatment, along with radiation for my brain tumors. Sunny also found me an integrative oncologist, and he did lots of IVs to help treat upstream. I also radically changed my diet.

Sunny told me that remission was not enough, that the cancer would come back if I did not clear up my biological terrain. She arranged a trip for me to see Dr. Yu in St. Louis. It was quite a journey, as my doctor said I could not fly due to brain swelling from the radiation. We took a 3-day Amtrak train each way.

Acupuncture meridian testing revealed several problems, including parasites, fungal, and dental – three root canals, #13, 18 and 31, along the meridians that were draining toxins into my lungs. I was referred to biological dentist Dr. Michael Rehme and had the infected teeth removed on an emergency basis. I was also advised to redo two crowns and have surgery to clean out two cavitations, work that began nearer my home.

Dr. Yu prescribed three cycles of antiparasitic and antifungal medications, along with oil pulling and homeopathic remedies. We also changed our diets. Sunny, my doctors and I were stunned when my scans – which first lit up like a Christmas tree, followed by shrinkage of my tumors with afatinib – now showed no signs of cancer, only some scar tissue. I will do additional rounds of medications, and then chelation to reduce high levels of mercury, lead and other heavy metals.

I am very fortunate. God gave me the best gift, my wife. For three years before my diagnosis, she had been exploring all the modalities. That informed her in helping me in the biggest fight of my life – and of the underlying problems I might have. Remission is great, but the cells are still there and can come back. They come back because you still have fundamental problems. Nobody but God knows. This is where you stop asking your oncologist – they don't know.

Learning the truth about health problems underlying many cancers, Sunny's intuition, and God's will are the factors I credit in my recovery journey. Dr. Yu is helping me tap into the magic of God. He is not just a doctor, but a healer. He doesn't just have knowledge, but wisdom. He is an instrument for diagnosis and healing; he gets to the bottom of things and gives you his wisdom.

Selected Articles on Cancer

Following are some of my articles on chronic inflammation and cancer, insulin potentiation therapy (IPT) to more effectively deliver low-dose drug therapy and nutritional supplements, ivermectin as an antiparasitic anticancer treatment, and cancer as a metabolic disease, for those who would like more background. While some parts are technical, they also contain information on dietary approaches that can be helpful during cancer treatment.

Article: Parasites, Inflammation and Cancer: Ring of Fire Feeding Tumor Cells

Cancer doesn't always originate where you think it does. Here are some surprising insights about how infectious microbes and inflammation lead to cancer.

"Chronic inflammation" is a new catch phrase for the explanation of all chronic degenerative diseases from asthma, arthritis, heart diseases, and irritable bowel disease to cancers. Unrecognized low-grade infection is one of the main culprits causing chronic inflammation. The link between infection and cancer has been recognized for many years and reported by many medical practitioners. However, it has never been widely accepted by medical authorities due to a lack of reliable, reproducible data to support this observation – until now.

A missing link in the relationship between infection, inflammation, and cancer was finally provided by the brilliant, groundbreaking research on stem cells done by Jean Marie Houghton, MD, PhD at the University of Massachusetts Medical School. Her work, specifically related to the formation of stomach cancer, first published in 2004, showed a cause-and-effect relationship between bacterial infection and cancer. In addition, she showed that this relationship is hidden under the disguise of chronic inflammation.[43] Her work led to an understanding that all forms of **infectious microbes**, including viruses, bacteria, and parasites, can create an **inflammatory immune response** which, under toxic environmental conditions, can cause cancer cells to grow.

Specifically, she showed that stomach cancer originates from bone marrow-derived cells, not from stomach lining cells as expected. Bone marrow-derived stem cells have "cancer-like properties." These properties include the capacity for unlimited growth, the ability to avoid programmed cell death signals, and the capacity to develop into many tissue types.

A process must occur in order for the bone marrow-derived stem cells to transform into cancer. First, chronic inflammation created by a pre-existing bacterial infection, such as Helicobacter pylori (H. pylori), damages the stomach lining. This creates a need for the influx of bone marrow-derived stem cells to migrate to the stomach. The stem cells migrate to the stomach specifically for the repair of the stomach lining by actually transforming themselves into stomach lining cells.

Next, once the stem cells are in the stomach, they are under undesirable influences from the inflammation itself, as well as synthetic hormones, viruses, some bacteria, parasites, and environmental toxins such as heavy metals and chemicals. These influences can cause stem cells to transform into cancer cells rather than stomach cells. **Reread these last three paragraphs: they are crucial to understanding the process of cancer cell creation.**

Some other major sources of chronic inflammation to consider include: hidden dental infections, old trauma, ulcerative colitis, Crohn's disease, chronic allergies, overtraining in athletes, electromagnetic stimulation, and unresolved emotional trauma. These multiple sources of inflammation create a "ring of fire" in our body. This "ring of fire" causes our immune system to burn out and lose control, which then allows cancer cells to evade our weakened immune surveillance and proliferate.

Therefore, due to the complexity of the behavior and biology of cancer cells, rather than micromanage the biochemistry of the cancer cells as in conventional treatments, our primary focus should be on detecting and eliminating the sources of inflammation. In particular, eradicating hidden infections should be one of the highest priorities for all cancer patients. Infections may come from viruses, parasites, and root canal dental infections. They can also be hidden in many different parts of organs and different layers of tissues.

Eradicating infections and inflammation should be combined with cleansing and detoxification of internal toxins and nutritional support for the body to heal. Detoxification and nutritional support are the best preventive actions to reduce the cancer risk factors mentioned above. Some well-known nutritional supports include: curcumin, mushroom extracts, lactoferrin, beta glucans, vitamin C, vitamin D, bioflavonoids, green tea extracts, and Essiac tea. Most of these nutrients can reduce inflammation, slow angiogenesis and metastasis, and boost immune functions. For more details, see the article on my website titled "Nutritional Therapies for Cancer."

For quite some time, cancer has been the second leading cause of death in the United States after heart attack and cardiovascular-related disease. Cancer will become the leading cause of death soon unless we make a dramatic change in our understanding and treatment of the causes and effects of chronic inflammation.

Medical science has been focusing on molecular biology. It's been targeting cancer cells with a "magic bullet" drug delivery system. In an ideal world, new understanding of the cause of inflammation and the "ring of fire" should shift the paradigm of medical science to a new way of diagnosing and treating infectious microbes.

Article: Insulin Potentiation Therapy (IPT)

Targeted low-dose therapies, accompanied by insulin to starve cancer cells, provide a tool to combat cancer. This is equivalent to a Trojan horse, bringing the soldiers to the enemy's well-protected cancer cells.

Insulin has been known to the medical community and the public primarily for the management of diabetes. However, is there an indication for using insulin therapy for conditions other than diabetes? I didn't recognize its full potential until I attended the IPT conference in Dallas in April 2012.

Insulin was first discovered by a Canadian medical doctor, Dr. Frederick Banton, and a medical student, Charles Best, in 1921. Before insulin was available, diabetes mellitus was a rare but deadly disease. Dr. Banton won the Nobel Prize in Medicine in 1923 with his professor John Macleod at the University of Toronto for their achievement in discovering insulin. Charles Best, the medical student, was not recognized for his work.

Soon after the discovery of insulin, Eli Lilly started large-scale production of insulin extract. Since then, insulin therapy has been a main therapeutic agent for insulin-dependent diabetes and type II diabetes. Although insulin doesn't cure diabetes, it has saved countless lives of diabetic patients. It is considered one of the most significant discoveries and successes of modern medicine.

Insulin has been tried for other medical conditions without much success in the U.S. Insulin Shock Therapy was tried by psychiatrists for severe depression without significant results or further development. This technique eventually lost interest with advancement in psychiatric medications. Most people only know insulin is for diabetes. Its use for other medical conditions has been mostly ignored.

In 1932, in Mexico, insulin potentiation therapy (IPT), a new game-changer in medicine, was conceived by a Mexican military surgeon, Donato Perez Garcia, Sr., MD. There were many documented cases of recoveries from asthma, psoriasis, migraines, vascular headaches, rheumatoid arthritis, intoxications, slipped disc, hemiplegia, multiple sclerosis, lupus, allergies, circulation problems, and even cancers.

What is IPT? Why was this therapy ignored for 80 years? Perhaps it was because it seems too simple and is hard to believe for all its claims. I had a hard time believing in IPT when I heard about it for the first time around 2002. Dr. Donato Garcia's first use of IPT was in the successful treatment of tertiary neurosyphilis. In 1944, *Time Magazine* covered the story of Dr. Garcia's IPT. They called his therapy Insulin Shock Treatment. Despite coverage by major media, his idea was never accepted in the United States. IPT was too simple of an idea. It was hard to believe it cured all sorts of chronic diseases. There was also a bias and prejudice against the Mexican medical profession, combined with the influence of pharmaceutical companies that didn't want such a simple cure.

IPT is truly a simple therapy. Give regular insulin (calculated based on body weight) intravenously to bring sugar levels into the range of 40-50 or when the patient is having hypoglycemic symptoms (sweating, increase in pulse, some sense of dizziness or weakness), then infuse dextrose to reverse the hypoglycemia. That is it. During the episode of hypoglycemia, the physician can infuse small amounts of specific medications for that particular medical condition. The dose of the medication can be reduced to 10% of the regular dose. It is still as highly effective as the standard dose of medications with minimum side effects.

Dr. Donato Garcia has been treating every known chronic disease with IPT, and he eventually started treating cancer. Cancer cells have a unique and characteristic cell membrane, with six times more insulin receptors and 10 times more IGF (insulin growth factor) receptors per cell than normal host cell membranes. As a result, cancer cells devour glucose better than normal cells.

IPT utilizes insulin to deliberately induce a hypoglycemic state to starve the cancer cells. However, during the state of hypoglycemia, the starving cancer cells are given low-dose chemotherapy agents or natural anti-cancer substances immediately followed by dextrose sugar. The low-dose chemotherapy agents are therefore devoured by and readily absorbed into the cancer cells.

Cancer cells are absorbing the sugar-chemotherapy agent solution before it gets to normal cells. Therefore, normal cells are minimally affected by low-dose chemotherapy therapy. IPT is equivalent to a **Trojan horse** that **brings the soldiers (remedies) to only the enemy's well-protected cancer cells.**

There are small groups of American medical doctors practicing IPT. They are trying to promote IPT as a safer and cheaper alternative to high-dose chemotherapy therapy and to train other doctors. I completed four days of training in IPT. The most exciting part of IPT is that it does not have to use low-dose chemotherapy to be effective. Dr. Donato Garcia successfully treated cancer without using any medications. Also, natural substances can be used without using chemotherapy agents.

It is time to honestly reassess the "War on Cancer" and look for more options. For more information, contact International Organization of Integrative Cancer Physicians (IOICP), or do a Google search on insulin potentiation therapy (IPT) or Best Answer for Cancer Foundation. The Cancer Control Society is another organization promoting safer integrative cancer therapies to medical professionals and the public.

Article: Ivermectin Deficiency Syndrome

Ivermectin deworming medicine is commonly prescribed by veterinarians, but it may be able to clear up medically unexplained symptoms (MUS) and some cancers.

A small group of researchers are racing to find a new cure for cancer from forgotten old medications. One of the medications is ivermectin, a common parasite medication used for dogs as a heart worm medication. Most veterinarians recommend deworming dogs with monthly ivermectin as a preventive measure.

Have you had ivermectin lately? If you have medically unexplainable symptoms (MUS) or cancer, you may consider trying ivermectin. Talk to your doctor, although unfortunately, most medical doctors are not familiar with the hidden epidemic of parasite problems and/or the usage of parasite medications.

Ivermectin is an old parasite medication isolated in 1979 and widely used since the 1980s for dogs, horses, and humans. Ivermectin is exceptionally potent. It is a broad spectrum antiparasitic drug which kills nematodes like pinworm,

Strongyloides, Ascaris, and Onchocerca. In fact, ivermectin is one of my favorite and most frequently used parasite medications.

Ivermectin selectively blocks the worm's GABA receptors but not the mammalian counterpart. It is a muscle relaxant which blocks the phosphorylation of the Ascaris muscle. Often, I will combine ivermectin with pyrantel pamoate, praziquantel, or tinidazole for a variety of medically unexplained symptoms.

I have experienced some dramatic responses for medically unexplained symptoms and some cancer cases using ivermectin and other antiparasitic medications. The selection of medications and dosages is guided by Acupuncture Meridian Assessment.

I have presented my case studies at a range of medical conferences. A physician who heard my lecture told me that ivermectin has anticancer and anticancer stem cell properties.

At a higher dose, ivermectin can inactivate the protein kinase PAK1 and blocks the PAK1-dependent growth of human ovarian cancer and neurofibromatosis Type 2 (NF2) tumor cell lines.[44] PAK proteins encoded by the PAK1 gene are critical for cytoskeleton reorganization and nuclear signaling.

This is probably more than you want to know about this parasite medication unless you have an unusual medical condition or cancer. PAK1 kinase is required for the growth of more than 70% of human cancers, such as pancreatic, colon, breast and prostate cancers, and neurofibromatosis.

The p21-activated kinase PAK1 is implicated in tumor genesis. Inhibiting PAK1 signals induces tumor cell apoptosis (cell death). PAK1 has also been implicated for maintenance of glucose homeostasis in pancreatic beta cells and skeletal muscle.[45]

Sumaiya Sharmeen et al. published research in the journal *Blood* that indicates ivermectin induces chloride-dependent membrane hyperpolarization and cell death in leukemia cells.[46] The paper states ivermectin synergizes with chemotherapeutic agents cytarabine and daunorubicin to induce cell death in leukemia cells.

This research shows that using a chemotherapeutic agent with a deworming medication can make chemotherapy more effective for chemotherapy-resistant leukemia. Cancer stem cells are the reason why cancer cells often develop resistance to chemotherapies. Research is telling us that a combination of chemotherapeutic agents and ivermectin is targeting cancer stem cells. Killing cancer stem cells is the holy grail of cancer therapy.

The story does not end with ivermectin. Zhen Hua Wu et al. published in *PLOS One* that praziquantel, my other favorite parasite medication for liver flukes, synergistically enhances paclitaxel (Taxol) efficacy to inhibit cancer cell growth.[47] Taxol is a common chemotherapeutic agent for ovarian cancer, breast cancer, small cell lung cancer, head and neck cancer, esophageal cancer, prostate and bladder cancer.

The clinical data indicate that praziquantel could greatly enhance the anticancer efficacy of Taxol in various cell lines, including Taxol-resistant cell lines. The combined treatment induced significant mitotic arrest and activated apoptotic cascades resulting in tumor cell death. The concept of a new use for an old drug is not a new idea, but there is not much financial incentive for pharmaceutical companies.

You wonder how many old forgotten medications are available in your pharmacy's medicine cabinet. The search for an old new cure continues by a small group of researchers. This research is one of the latest new trends.

Once this information gets out into mainstream medicine, I wonder if they will create an "ivermectin deficiency syndrome." Monthly deworming for medically unexplained symptoms or for cancer patients might be a better solution than searching for this mysterious ivermectin deficiency syndrome.

Article: Searching for an Old New Cure: Update on Parasite Medications

Recently, one of the compound pharmacists shared that that they now have a hard time getting ivermectin, and recommended using different parasite medications. Ivermectin also has very strong anti-cancer properties, which I wrote about in my previous article, "Ivermectin Deficiency Syndrome." At high doses, ivermectin can inactivate the protein kinase PAK-1, and block the PAK-1 dependent growth of human ovarian cancer and neurofibromatosis type 2 (NF2) tumors. PAK-1 kinase is required for the growth of more than 70% of human cancers such as pancreatic, colon, breast prostate, and NF2 cancers.

When I was at Medicine Week 2018 in Germany, I gave a talk on Parasite Medications for Targeting Cancer. Dr. Helmut Retzek, MD of Austria told me about using niclosamide with great success on a pancreatic cancer patient at Dr. med. Friedrich Douwes' St. George Clinic in Bad Aibling, Germany. He shared an article from the *Chinese Journal of Cancer*, "Niclosamide, an old anthelminthic agent, demonstrating antitumor activity by blocking multiple signaling pathways of cancer stem cells."[48]

The activity of niclosamide against parasites (tapeworm and schistosomiasis) is believed to be mediated by inhibition of mitochondrial oxidative phosphorylation and anaerobic ATP production. Niclosamide targets multiple signaling pathways (NF-kB, Wnt/B-catenin, Notch, ROS, mTOR1 and Stat3), most of which are closely involved with cancer stem cells. Niclosamide has shown anti-proliferative activity in a broad spectrum of cancer cells, such as acute myeloid leukemia, colon, breast and prostate cancer. This medication has been available for the last 50 years and is virtually unknown to oncologists.

Suramin was introduced in Germany in 1920, nearly a century ago, for treatment of the protozoal parasite Trypanosoma, which causes African sleeping sickness. Suramin is also used against retroviruses by inhibiting retroviral reverse transcriptase and blocking the binding of various growth factors, such as insulin-like growth factor (IGF-1), epidermal growth factor (EGF), platelet-derived growth factor (PDGF), transforming growth factor-beta (TGF-beta), vascular endothelial growth factor (VEGF), and basic fibroblast growth factor (bFGF). It induces angiogenesis with apparent anti-cancer effects. Suramin can only be given intravenously and I have not yet tried it. In the United States, Suramin is available only from the CDC Drug Service; one cannot get it from compounding pharmacies. Suramin has been reported to be used with success with some autistic children. I wrote about connections on parasites and autism in, "Medical Acupuncture on Gallbladder Meridian: Therapeutic Illusion on IBS and Autism," in Chapter 5.

These older medications that kill parasites in the body also have anticancer properties, unknown to most physicians. Interestingly, cancer behaves as if cancer is a metabolic parasite. You may wonder what else we are missing and why we are blinded from this important medical information, hidden and buried right in front of our eyes. Any medications can be used off-label; are they not utilized because of our ignorance, or because there is no money to be made in using older medications for other indications? Albendazole and mebendazole, developed in the 1970s for pinworms, are on WHO's Essential Medicines list. Albendazole costs pennies in low-income countries, a few dollars in nations like the UK; in the U.S., up to $400 per dose (two pills).

If this information becomes more widely accepted by physicians, oncologists, hospitals, and academic medical schools, there will be a major shock wave at the core of our medical education system and medicine itself. Parasites are also embedded in the brain as well as in our teeth/jaw/root canals and parasites might be the driving force, at the top of the food chain in the Evolution of Life. Perhaps, we are deliberately misled and ignore this information because, as I like to say, "Big pharma became the dominant parasite - metaphorically." How can we counter attack and break the cycle of the parasites?

Article: Cancer as a Metabolic Disease as if Cancer is Metabolic Parasites

Cancer cells rely on glucose (anaerobic glycolysis fermentation) as the predominant source of energy for survival. This is often referred to as the Warburg effect. Thomas Seyfried's book is a groundbreaking new approach to understanding and treating cancer based on Dr. Otto Warburg's work and the ketogenic diet.

Thomas N. Seyfried's book, *Cancer as a Metabolic Disease: On the Origin, Management, and Prevention of Cancer*, is a seminal work. As noted by its publisher Wiley, "The book addresses controversies related to the origins of cancer and provides solutions to cancer management and prevention. It expands upon Otto Warburg's well-known theory that all cancer is a disease of energy metabolism."

The latest scientific studies indicate that the ketogenic diet can also be used effectively as a complementary cancer therapy with a new understanding of the metabolism of cancer cells. This section draws on Thomas Seyfried, PhD's idea of the ketogenic diet as a main nutritional therapy for cancer management based on science and biochemistry.

All cancer cells rely on glucose (glycolysis fermentation) as the predominant source of energy for survival. This is often referred to as the Warburg effect. Seyfried's book is a groundbreaking new approach to understanding and treating cancer based on Dr. Otto Warburg's effect and the ketogenic diet. If you have or had cancer, you need to read his book. It may save your life.

Otto Warburg won the Nobel Prize in 1931 for his discovery of oxygen-transferring enzymes and the mode of action of the respiratory enzyme. He was nominated for a second Nobel Prize for his work on nicotinamide and discovering flavin (the yellow enzyme), but it was denied by Adolf Hitler's Nazi regime. His most important work was on cancer cell metabolism. Warburg proved that aerobic glycolysis fermentation is the hallmark of cancer regardless of the tissue origin. Glycolysis is the first stop in the breakdown of glucose – sugar – to extract energy for cellular metabolism. Warburg's work was challenged, dismissed, and forgotten by mainstream medical academic institutions.

Some medical doctors have tried to bring his ideas back into the mainstream by applying a low-carb/low-sugar diet. This diet mimics the ketogenic diet to curb the growth of tumors. This met with limited acceptance and success, as mainstream medicine did not fully understand how a ketogenic diet affects the metabolism of cancer cells. Chemotherapy, radiation, and surgery became the mainstream therapy for cancer management for the last 60 years.

If I mention the ketogenic diet to my patients, most of them have no idea what I'm talking about. They think it is too medically esoteric for them to understand or they are terrorized with a gruesome dangerous starvation diet. Fasting is the fastest way to go into the ketogenic state but fasting does not mean starvation. I previously wrote an article, "40-Day Fast for Parasite Eradication." A 40-day fast is the ultimate ketogenic diet.

Metabolically, cancer behaves like metabolic parasites according to Dr. Tim Guilford, MD. He presented a lecture on glutathione, cancer, and the Warburg effect at the 8th International Integrative Medical Conference in St. Louis. People are always looking for a new diet as a new cure. If you get tired of hearing of the ketogenic diet and are looking for an exotic fancy diet, how about we modify the name "ketogenic diet" and call it the Genghis Khan diet? Genghis Khan Diet is battle proven, starving and terrorizing the enemy called cancer: metabolic parasite.

Thomas Seyfried's book extensively covers the metabolic management of cancer with the ketogenic diet. His book is technical with lots of biochemistry and not an easy to book to read. For the general public, you may want to start with *The Cantin Ketogenic Diet*, by Elaine Cantin.

Dr. Seyfried goes much more in depth on the origin, management, and prevention of cancer. Read his book. It may save your life. Highlights of its major conclusions include:

1. No real progress has been made in the management of advanced or metastatic cancer for more than 40 years.

2. Most of the conceptual advances made in understanding the mechanisms of cancer have more to do with non-metastatic tumors than metastatic tumors.

3. Most cancer, regardless of cell or tissue origin, is a singular disease of respiratory insufficiency coupled with compensatory glycolysis fermentation as a primary cause of cancer.

4. Secondary causes of cancer include age, viral infection, hypoxia, inflammation, rare inherited mutations, radiation, and carcinogens.

5. Genomic instability seen in tumors is a downstream epiphenomenon and makes cancer cells vulnerable to metabolic stress.

6. Cancer cells do not have a growth advantage over normal cells.

7. Cancer progression is not Darwinian but Lamarckian.

8. Most cancer is not a genetic disease. Therefore, gene research into the causes of cancer is no longer credible.

9. Respiratory injury can explain Szent-Gyorgyi's oncogenic paradox: that a very specific process could be initiated in very unspecific ways.

10. Most metastatic cancers arise from respiratory injury in the myeloid origin of macrophages.

11. Cancer cells depend on glucose and glutamine metabolism for survival and growth.

12. Restricted access to glucose and glutamine will compromise cancer cell growth and survival.

13. Enhanced glycolysis fermentation is largely responsible for tumor cell drug resistance.

14. Protection of mitochondria from oxidative damage will prevent or reduce risk of cancer.

15. Lifestyle changes will be needed to manage and prevent cancer.

16. Mitochondrial-enhancement therapies, administered together with drugs that target glucose and glutamine metabolism, will go far as a nontoxic, cost-effective solution to the cancer problem.

17. A new era for cancer management and prevention will emerge once cancer becomes recognized as a metabolic disease.

Article: Cancer is an Infectious Disease as if Cancer is Metabolic Parasites: Biology of Cancer Cells

New research demonstrates that antibiotics that target mitochondria effectively eradicate cancer stem cells, across multiple tumor types: treating cancer like an infectious disease. There is an Achilles' heel in cancer stem cells' mitochondria: because of their evolution eons ago, cancer mitochondria are more susceptible to classes of mitochondria-targeted antibiotics.

Dr. Tim Guilford, MD from California emailed me a Research Paper Review article by Rebecca Lamb et al. from *Oncotarget* titled, "Antibiotics that target mitochondria effectively eradicate cancer stem cells, across multiple tumor types: treating cancer like an infectious disease."[49] This research paper, published in January 2015, came from and received startup funding from the University of Manchester, England. It proposed to treat cancer like an infectious disease by using FDA-approved antibiotics as anti-cancer therapy, across multiple tumor types.

The research paper proposed a new strategy for the treatment of early cancerous lesions and advanced metastatic disease, via selective targeting of cancer stem cells, also known as tumor-initiating cells, by utilizing well-known antibiotics. The clinical practice of targeting genetic mutation and gene therapy has been disappointing, in that cancer control has been short-lived, even when these gene-targeted drugs are proven to be effective in clinical trials.

Based on their study, 4-5 different classes of FDA-approved antibiotics can be used to eradicate cancer stem cells, in 12 different cancer cell lines, across eight different tumor types, including breast, ductal carcinoma in situ (DCIS), ovarian, prostate, melanoma, and glioblastoma of the brain. Those classes of mitochondria-targeted antibiotics include: erythromycin-azithromycin, tetracycline-doxycycline, glycylcyclines, and an antiparasitic drug, pyrvinium pamoate, and chloramphenicol. Pyrvinium pamoate is not commercially available in the U.S., and one may use pyrantel pamoate or combine with ivermectin.

Dr. Tim Guilford coined the phrase "cancer is metabolic parasites" at the 8th St. Louis Integrative Integrative Medicine Conference in 2013. I have written many articles in connection with hidden parasite infections, inflammation, and development of tumor cells. In fact, cancer cells behave very much like metabolic parasites, taking energy away from the host. Sometimes tumors disappear with parasite medications.

The crux of the hypothesis is based on understanding the **Achilles' heel** in cancer stem cells' mitochondria. Because mitochondria evolved from bacteria that were originally engulfed by early eukaryotic-protozoa cells over one billion years ago (known as the endosymbiotic theory of mitochondrial evolution), **cancer mitochondria are more susceptible to classes of mitochondria-targeted antibiotics.**

Mitochondrial biogenesis – the production of new living organisms or organelles – is required for the propagation of all cancer stem cells. Bacterial and cancer cells' mitochondrial large (50S) and small (30S) ribosomes are similar in size and function. They are susceptible to antibiotics which target mitochondrial biogenesis and eradicate cancer stem cells with manageable side effects.

In essence, we can treat cancer not based on genetic mutations, but based on a common global mitochondrial phenotypic property that is characteristic of cancer stem cells. This applies to many cancer types. Importantly, azithromycin, tigecycline, and doxycycline are known to cross the blood-brain barrier, making the treatment of brain cancer with these antibiotics feasible.

Their hypothesis of mitochondrial biogenesis of cancer stem cells is similar to, if not consistent with, Otto Warburg's theory of cancer as a metabolic disease. This is because all cancer cells rely on glucose (glycolysis fermentation) as the predominant source of energy for their survival (the Warburg effect). As noted in the previous article, *Cancer is a Metabolic Disease,* by Thomas Seyfried, PhD, eloquently explains this understanding and how to treat cancer based on the Warburg effect and ketogenic diet.

Eukaryotic protozoa cells evolved from our universal ancestor a billion years ago, incorporating endo-symbiotic bacteria as mitochondrial cellular power plants. Human cells are a product of the creation and biological evolution of eukaryotic protozoa cells.

When our physical body is fed a faulty diet, including processed and genetically altered food, lives in toxic environments, lives with chronic infections, and when we are under constant attack with fear and toxic emotions, our body starts to degenerate. It may manifest as diabetes, heart problems, autoimmune disease, arthritis, or tumors as our bodies become more acidic and toxic.

Cancer is a form of the biological degeneration of our survival mechanism when our trillions of cells are not living in harmony. It becomes metabolically similar to protozoal mitochondria, surviving on glycolysis fermentation, due to respiratory insufficiency of mitochondria as predicted by Otto Warburg.

Is it possible to reverse the process of cancerous conditions? It takes more than antibiotics or antiparasitic medications to treat cancer. We need to treat the whole body on physical, emotional, and spiritual levels.

However, based on these well researched papers, it is worthwhile to start using natural and prescribed antibiotics, antifungal, and antiparasitic medications as a means to reduce the total burden of infections, as a part of cancer management programs by primary care physicians. It may have a secondary benefit of targeting the mitochondria of cancer stem cells. This research paper gives us a glimpse of hope and the possibility of a cure for cancer.

Chapter 10 Lyme and Persistent Lyme

*Can we solve the mystery of persistent Lyme
by applying the analogy of forensic science?
Who committed the crime of persistent Lyme?*

Introduction to Lyme and Persistent Lyme

Lyme disease and especially, chronic, persistent, or resistant Lyme continue to cause misery for many and confound practitioners on how best to treat it. The latest medical hypothesis indicates that Lyme disease is linked to over 300 diseases, including fibromyalgia, chronic fatigue syndrome, Parkinson's disease, MS, ALS, brain fog, dilated cardiomyopathy, anxiety, and a wide spectrum of physical and psychiatric dysfunctions. The CDC calls it post-treatment Lyme disease syndrome (PTLDS), assuming all antibiotics work and all patients recover, which patients rightly find wrong and dismissive. Nobody says patients have post-cancer.

In my experience, patients with persistent Lyme often have multiple, overlapping problems that need to be addressed, including parasites, fungal, dental, heavy metals, and nutritional problems, in addition to the Lyme bacterium. Patients may think they only have one disease, while there are many problems to be addressed, in addition to Lyme and co-infections.

There are many comprehensive resources on Lyme disease and persistent Lyme, so I will not discuss the basics here. Readers may consider Richard I. Horowitz, MD's books, including *Why Can't I Get Better? Solving the Mystery of Lyme & Chronic Disease*

(2013) and, *How Can I Get Better? An Action Plan for Treating Resistant Lyme and Chronic Disease* (2017).

Horowitz introduces the concept of Multiple Systemic Infectious Disease Syndrome (MSIDS) to describe everything that can potentially go wrong because of Lyme and coinfections, and their impacts on the immune system and its ability to withstand or react to other infections, heavy metals, chemical toxins and mycotoxins. He presents a 16-point differential diagnostic map which outlines specific symptoms, possible related medical conditions, and laboratory tests to consider.

Another excellent book is Neil Nathan, MD's, *Toxic: Heal Your Body from Mold Toxicity, Lyme Disease, Multiple Chemical Sensitivities, and Chronic Environmental Illness* (2018). Both physicians examine the multiple, overlapping causes of Lyme-related chronic illnesses, and a wide range of treatment strategies to address them. Nathan uses the analogy of rebooting the many systems that break down in the body. I like this analogy. This paradigm can be further advanced by adding the energetic dimension via AMA, to gain information and intelligence to develop battle plans for a total systems reboot in the order and sequence needed.

Scott's Story: From Wrecked to Recovered

Scott Forsgren shares his Lyme journey and recovery quest for my book. Imagine you learn that "Lyme disease" is so much more, and that many stones must be uncovered to regain wellness.

Imagine a life where you seemingly have it all. Imagine wanting for nothing more, except for the continuance of your already blessed life. Actually, I never really wished for that as I always took it for granted.

Now imagine that almost overnight it is taken away. This is how it happened to me. It all began with what seemed like a viral infection, and in just a few short days had become a major illness which continued to baffle the best medicine had to offer for days, weeks, months, and even years. My life was forever changed.

Imagine the fear one feels when presented with the unknown. Imagine the isolation and the desperation that one might experience when being confronted with a serious, unknown illness that, at the time, felt as though it literally could have taken my life. Unfortunately, it does not take imagination to understand what this might feel like; for this had become what was left of me.

Imagine a constant burning sensation throughout your entire body that is at times almost unbearable. My body burned like someone had poured acid on it. Beyond the physical pain, there was the emotional pain which was generated by the uncertainty of what had become my existence.

Imagine having a fever that lasts for over a year, all the while having doctors and others trying to convince you that it might be "normal." In your heart, you know that this is far from normal, but you find it impossible to convince anyone that it is a sign of something gone seriously awry.

Imagine that you no longer have to imagine what it is like to feel sick day in and day out. Suddenly, it becomes you. You become it. Nothing else matters except the quest to return to your previous life. In fact, this was a new life filled with fear as well as physical and emotional pain unlike anything I had experienced in the past.

I remember it all so vividly from head to toe. Odd tingling sensations ran through my body. My vision was blurred more often than not. My ears were full of pressure and popped with every swallow.

Walking was a challenge due to the weak muscles in my legs. For several months, I could barely walk at all. Of course, that fueled my fears that I had a serious neurological disease. Simpler physical acts were also surprisingly difficult. Sitting in a chair proved challenging as my balance was off. I constantly felt as though I was falling to one side. No matter how much I propped myself up, the falling feeling never went away. I always felt as though I was going to roll off the bed and land on the floor.

Every muscle in my body was sore and every joint even sorer. I cannot count the nights that I cried myself to sleep due to the intense pain. It seemed to get worse as time went on, and I knew that the illness was progressing and the need for answers grew stronger and stronger each day. I would stare at my hands and feet, feel the pain, and wonder what it was that was causing it. It was undoubtedly the biggest mystery I would be faced with in my life, and I set my sights on solving it.

I had muscle twitches throughout my body. Eventually, almost every muscle in my body would at one time or another have these annoying little reminders that something was wrong.

My stomach was an entire set of problems and symptoms in and of itself. It hurt all the time. There was an intense burning that never seemed to end. If there was a list of GI symptoms that one could have, I certainly had almost all of them.

Imagine a motor-like, tapping sensation felt continuously in your arms, legs, and feet. Twenty-four hours a day, I felt this constant tapping sensation. Imagine that every doctor to whom you described this sensation looked at you with a blank stare as if to say they had no idea what was causing the problem; or if the problem was even real.

Imagine the day that you open a book which describes a "motor-like" sensation as a symptom of something called "Chronic Fatigue Syndrome." Imagine you search the Internet to find information on CFS which states that, *"The illness varies greatly in its duration. A few recover after a year or two. More often, those who recover are more likely to do so from 3 to 6 years after onset. Others may recover after a decade or more. Yet for some, the illness seems to simply persist."*

Great, so now I had a disease which had no known cause or origin, no known cure, and even worse, it could last for decades. Oh, the fear and desperation that I felt, and yet, I could think of nothing more than to continue the quest to research and figure out how to get myself out of this situation. I was certainly not giving up!

Imagine that one day you find out that the cause of your unexplained illness is actually "Lyme disease" and all of its not-so-delicious trimmings. Imagine that you find doctors that specialize in your particular illness and become your biggest mentors and influencers as you now have something tangible to work with. Imagine that you work hard over the next several years to make a comeback. It takes work, hard work. You struggle. You sacrifice. You listen, not only to your doctors, but to your own body and your inner-wisdom.

Imagine that you learn that "Lyme disease" is so much more, and that many stones must be uncovered to regain wellness. When I first started down my "Lyme" recovery journey, I was certain that infections were the most important thing to address and that I could kill my way back to health. Then, I began to understand that toxicity was an important consideration. I put the emotional contributors last on the list at the time; even though I knew I could certainly benefit from some work in this realm.

Today, I see things exactly the opposite. Getting one's emotional health in order is a top priority. Feeling we deserve to be well and remediating any false beliefs is critical. Detoxification became a major area of focus, and as time progressed, infections became less and less of a consideration. I went from viewing infections, toxins, and emotions as my priorities to an understanding they were really emotions, toxins, and then infections.

I had to consider a number of new concepts such as how living in an environment with toxic mold impacts health, how parasites affect us, how electromagnetic fields add further stress to our already weakened bodies, the impact of diet on inflammation and immune health, and how other factors such as underlying dental cavitations contribute to the imbalances that we perceive as illness. The next several years became a process of removing stressful items while adding numerous health-promoting ones to shift the balance back to my favor. It was not easy, but it was so worth it.

Imagine that little by little you improve. It takes time. In fact, at times, the improvement seems so slow that you almost don't notice that you are still improving, but you are. Imagine that one day, you don't think of yourself as having an illness anymore.

Imagine that you learn so much from the struggle and gain so many unexpected gifts along the way that you never again look at life in the same way. Imagine that life is good and you feel at peace... at last you feel peace. Imagine you are well.

Now, this was at one time hard for me to imagine, but fortunately, it did not take imagination because this became my reality. In my wildest imagination, I could not have believed that I would ever have gotten back to the place that I am today; I have literally gone from wrecked to recovered. I am truly blessed and forever grateful.

Scott Forsgren, FDN-P, "Better Health Guy," worked with Dr. Simon Yu on parasites, heavy metals, food allergies, and dental cavitations in old wisdom teeth sockets. He ultimately discovered that while Lyme disease was part of his underlying condition, he needed to cast a much broader net to regain his health, illustrating many of the key concepts discussed in this book. Scott shares his blog, knowledge, and podcasts at Better Health Guy, on Facebook, and at many events.

New Research on Lyme and Parasite Connections

According to pathologist Alan B. MacDonald, MD, examination of autopsied brain tissues from patients who died of serious neurological conditions revealed that many tick-borne infections, such as Lyme disease, go undiagnosed and untreated. He found two Borrelia pathogens, including B. burgdorferi, which causes Lyme disease, thriving inside parasitic nematode worms, worm eggs, or larvae in the brain tissue of 19 deceased patients. "Both the worms and the Borrelia pathogens can cause devastating brain damage," according to MacDonald. "Current tests, like the ELISA and Western blot, do not adequately detect the presence of Borrelia bacteria."[50] You can learn more about his research on his website, https://alzheimerborreliosis.net/research/.

Lyme is a spirochete, and other spirochetes also play a role in chronic immune and neurological illnesses and brain pathology. The most well-known in human history is syphilis. Other spirochetes include Treponema and Leptospira.

Article: Who Else Committed the Crime of Post-Lyme? Forensic Case Study from New York

I use the term Post-Lyme here on purpose, to be provocative. Sharon, a college professor from upstate New York and a classic persistent Lyme patient, provides a forensic case study. After myriad doctors and treatments, including lengthy IV antibiotics, IPT which led to pancreatitis, and major dental work, she came to see me for parasites and fungi, her missing link.

Who else committed the crime of Post-Lyme? The Integrative Medicine for the Treatment of Tick-borne Diseases Conference was held in Baltimore in April 2018, and the Lyme Disease Association of Delmarva invited me to give a talk. I told them I do not treat Lyme disease, I am not Lyme-literate, nor am I specialized in Lyme disease or tick-borne diseases. They may not have liked what I had to say, and may have asked the wrong person to give a talk. I do not see lots of Lyme patients as typically they will see a Lyme specialist and come only if treatment isn't helping.

The Association asked me to give a lecture on parasites in the context of Lyme and tick-borne diseases. I told them I am not a parasitologist but have written many articles on parasites based on my military experience. As long as they understand that, I would give a lecture on parasites, but also on hidden dental infections that can mimic Lyme disease.

There is a clear indication to use antibiotics for acute tick bite incidents with associated classic skin lesion of a bull's eye red rash and/or arthralgia and flu-like symptoms after a tick bite. What happens when the symptoms become progressive and develop into even more weird symptoms after antibiotics? Using more powerful antibiotics may not solve the problem.

There is great controversy in the area of Lyme when symptoms persist after treatment, or when diagnosis and treatment is missed. This is called post-treatment Lyme disease syndrome (PTLDS) by the U.S. Centers for Disease Control and Prevention (CDC) and the Infectious Disease Society of America (IDSA). In contrast, it is called persistent, resistant or chronic Lyme disease by most patients, and by International Lyme and Associated Diseases Society (ILADS) physicians.

If the Borrelia burgdorferi spirochete (Lyme) and co-infections are treated with aggressive IV antibiotics and the patient still has symptoms of Lyme, can we solve the mystery of Lyme by applying the analogy of forensic science? Let us investigate what happened after aggressively eliminating the Borrelia spirochete infection. In other words, who else committed the crime?

Forensic science is the application of science to criminal and civil laws, mainly during criminal investigation, as governed by the legal standards of **admissible evidence**. Assuming the Borrelia is dead, mutated, transformed, or hiding in cyst form, Lyme specialists look for co-infections as a culprit for persistent antibiotic Lyme symptoms, like Babesia, Bartonella, Ehrlichia, Anaplasma, Mycoplasma, and Rocky Mountain spotted fever. There may be other factors as well, overlapping and synergistic.

Let me introduce 60-year-old Sharon, a college professor from upstate New York and a classic Lyme syndrome patient, as a forensic case study. Sharon had a tick bite in 2013 and was on doxycycline and initially felt better. In 2014, she was told she had seronegative Lyme disease. In 2016, she experienced vision loss with white clouding on her vision, but the eye exam was normal. Since then, she experienced right eye pain and pins-and-needles-like pain, and has seen 13 physicians. She needs to use an eye patch to read, but her eye exam has been completely normal per numerous ophthalmologists.

A spinal tap was done in January 2017 and was positive for Borrelia. She was officially diagnosed with CNS neurologic Lyme disease. An infectious disease specialist started her on a 28-day course of IV ceftriaxone, and there was no improvement. She was told her Lyme disease was treated, and she now has post-Lyme syndrome. She experienced persistent tingling arms and legs, incontinence, lower back pain, fibromyalgia pain all over, severe fatigue, loss of appetite, weight loss, and severe insomnia.

The patient went to a Lyme clinic in Arizona and received a 10-week course of IV antibiotics and six weeks of insulin potentiation therapy (IPT), but developed pancreatitis during the course of treatment. Next she had oral surgery in Colorado for four cavitations and replacement of two amalgams, and "crashed" according to her words. She also had a coffee enema, during which she passed "two different kinds of parasites" – the admissible evidence – and came to see me for parasite problems.

Acupuncture Meridian Assessment (AMA) showed that 8 out of 40 meridians were out of balance. Her gallbladder, allergy/immunology, and small intestine meridians were the dominant problems. She was started on parasite meds: ivermectin, pyrantel pamoate, and praziquantel; followed by antifungal meds: fluconazole and itraconazole; and other support therapies.

On her second visit, she reported feeling much better, and all 40 meridians were balanced. She will be on multiple rounds of alternating parasite/antifungal meds. This is a long process of eliminating several layers of infections – including Borrelia burgdorferi and co-infections – with IV antibiotics, dental cavitation (jawbone) infections with oral surgery, and finally, parasites and fungal infections with potent prescribed medications.

It may be premature for me to say she is healing from persistent Lyme. Time will tell. From the forensic science of who committed the crime, her missing links between Lyme disease and "post-Lyme syndrome" were dental infections (four jawbone cavitations) and parasite/fungal infections.

Article: Lyme Disease, Autism and Beyond: Just Another New Fad or a New Modern Plague?

One of the hardest parts of my job is convincing patients to let go of the diagnosis of Lyme disease regardless of test results. They often have additional problems, including hidden dental infections from root canals, cavitations from old extracted tooth sockets, heavy metals, chronic allergies, and co-infections.

Lyme disease has been under the scrutiny of the medical community for overdiagnosis when the test does not meet all the criteria set by the Center for Disease Control (CDC) and the patient is prescribed an aggressive antibiotic treatment. Lyme disease seems to be one of the most overdiagnosed and also often misdiagnosed medical conditions.

Why is Lyme disease diagnosis controversial? The crux of the problem is the reliability of the laboratory test for Lyme disease. Lyme disease experts don't agree on the interpretation of the test results. I have addressed this critical issue in my article, "Lyme Disease Under the Limelight: Are the Diagnoses Misleading?"

In that article, I wrote I believe there are two distinctive diseases: Lyme disease caused by Borrelia burgdorferi and a Lyme disease-associated complex caused by many other underlying problems. Borrelia burgdorferi belongs to the spirochete family. One of the most famous diseases caused by spirochetes is not Lyme disease, but syphilis. Syphilis is caused by Treponema pallidum, a spirochete species. The other common spirochete infection comes from dental and periodontal disease and can cause carditis, neuropathy, arthralgia, fibromyalgia and severe fatigue – and can very much mimic Lyme disease caused by Borrelia burgdorferi.

Lyme disease patients often have co-infections with protozoa, from an intracellular red blood cell parasite called Babesia, and an intracellular bacterium, Ehrlichia. Missouri has a couple of Lyme disease specialists who treat aggressively with multiple oral and IV antibiotics along with antifungal medication. They have reported a great success rate for remission of Lyme disease.

The latest medical hypothesis indicates that Lyme disease is linked to over 300 diseases, including fibromyalgia, chronic fatigue syndrome, Parkinson's disease, MS, ALS, brain fog, dilated cardiomyopathy, anxiety, and a wide spectrum of physical and psychiatric dysfunctions including autism. The good news is that any stage of Lyme disease may respond to appropriate antibiotic treatment. Sometimes, the response can be dramatic.

I believe there are as many Lyme-like mimics and confounding overlapping causes of the disease complex as true Lyme disease. We need to differentiate and treat accordingly. Otherwise, once diagnosed with Lyme disease, patients may become victims of misdiagnosis or partial diagnosis, obsessed with Lyme disease, Borrelia infection and prolonged, multiple antibiotic therapies, including IV antibiotics.

One of the hardest parts of my job is convincing the patient to let go of the diagnosis of Lyme disease regardless of the test results. They often have more than Lyme disease. They may have significant hidden dental infections from root canals, cavitations from old extracted tooth sockets, heavy metal exposure, chronic allergies, and other parasite co-infections. Even when their symptoms respond by correcting dental infections and parasite problems, they still have a hard time letting go of the antibiotics. The antibiotics become their security blanket.

Dietrich Klinghardt, MD, PhD, a pioneer in the field of Integrative Medicine in Seattle, originally from Germany, specializes in Lyme disease and autism. He invited me to give a lecture on parasites at his conference, called A Deep Look Beyond Lyme, in May 2011. Two years prior to this event, I gave a lecture on parasites in Baden-Baden, Germany at the Medicine Week conference. I met Dr. Klinghardt and discussed some of the incurable medical problems caused by unrecognized parasite infections and how to treat them with appropriate medications.

He reported there has been a dramatically improved response rate in autistic children and Lyme disease patients when they were treated with antiparasitic medications before starting antibiotic usage. He even gave me credit for aggressively using parasite medications. He calls it, "modified Dr. Simon Yu's parasite protocol." The patient may not require many months or years of antibiotics, but only require a few weeks of antibiotics after the parasite medications.

I had the privilege to share my experience with about 150 medical professionals at the Seattle conference through my lecture titled, "Think Parasites and Dental When the Latest Medical Therapies Failed." Dr. Klinghardt recognized the key role of the missing link for improved response rates in autistic children and Lyme patients after treating their parasite infections. We became a team teaching how to treat hidden parasites. He uses ART (Autonomic Response Testing), and I use AMA (Acupuncture Meridian Assessment) to detect and treat parasites.

The conference was a great experience for me to learn more about autism and Lyme disease. There is a link between autism and hidden Lyme disease. Dr. Klinghardt reports that kryptopyrroluria (KPU) or hemopyrrollactamuria (HPU) is a major piece of the puzzle in overcoming chronic Lyme disease, as well as autism. For an overview, see "Kryptopyrroluria 2017: A Major Piece of the Puzzle in Overcoming Chronic Lyme Disease," by Scott Forsgren and Dietrich Klinghardt.[51]

HPU is a biomarker and neurotoxic substance frequently identified in the urine of patients with autism, learning disabilities, alcoholism, substance abuse, schizophrenia, ADHD, Down's syndrome, bipolar disorders, and even criminal behavior. The original study was done by a Canadian psychiatrist, Abram Hoffer, MD, PhD, the father of orthomolecular psychiatry, looking for the origin of schizophrenia.

Dr. Klinghardt also found an association with KPU and HPU for patients with heavy metal toxicity, autism, Lyme disease, multiple sclerosis, and Parkinson's. HPU levels can be measured from urine by Health Diagnostics and Research Institute's lab in the U.S. The crux of the problem might be that HPU in the urine is not a stable compound, and the test results may not be as reliable as the interpretation of the Lyme test.

What have I learned by attending his Seattle conference? Symptoms of Lyme disease and autism are the latest controversial medical conditions. They can be labeled as the latest fad and fit into MUS (medically unexplained symptoms) like chronic fatigue syndrome, fibromyalgia or irritable bowel syndrome. If we continue to ignore the true cause of the problems, Lyme disease and these other conditions may turn into new modern plagues.

Chapter 11 Extraordinary Patients and Unexplained Diseases

I told her that I was hoping that we were wearing helmets on the same team and not against each other. When I told her that, she calmed down.

Chronic diseases are on the rise, and conventional medicine does not have enough to offer patients who suffer from them. My inability to help such patients led me on my own journey to expand my knowledge, learn new tools, and develop more effective strategies and battle plans to treat them.

U.S. Statistics on Chronic Diseases and Deaths (CDC)

According to the Centers for Disease Control and Prevention (CDC), chronic diseases – heart disease and stroke, cancer, diabetes, chronic lung diseases, and others – account for most deaths in the United States and globally. Chronic diseases and conditions are the major drivers of sickness, disability, and healthcare costs in the nation.

The statistics are troubling: 60 percent of U.S. adults have a chronic disease and four in ten have two or more chronic health conditions.[52] Ninety percent of the nation's healthcare costs are spent on those with chronic and mental health conditions. The economic, social, family and personal costs are staggering.

- Heart disease and stroke comprise one-third of all deaths in the United States, over 810,000 per year.

- Cancer is the second leading cause of death. Each year, more than 1.7 million people are diagnosed with cancer, and almost 600,000 die from it.
- More than 29 million people have diabetes, and another 86 million adults have prediabetes, which puts them at risk.
- Obesity is a serious health concern, impacting more than one-third of adults, and one in five children. Over one in four Americans 17-24 years old are too heavy to join the military.
- Arthritis is the most common cause of disability. Of the 54 million adults with a doctor's diagnosis of arthritis, about 40% say they have trouble with usual daily activities because of their arthritis.
- Alzheimer's disease affects 5.7 million Americans. It is the sixth leading cause of death among all adults, and fifth for those aged 65 and older. [53]

Time to Unmask the Drug-Based Therapeutic Illusion

Too many patients are not getting better, and we do not have enough to offer them. Increasingly, our modern medical system is based on a lucrative, "drug-based therapeutic illusion" – a "pill culture" – created and fueled by global pharmaceutical companies. Ever since the United States became one of only two countries that allow direct-to-consumer drug advertising, TV shows, magazines, and the Internet have become saturated with alluring, compelling and seductive ads for the next new costly drugs. Typically, drugs for chronic diseases may alleviate symptoms, improve lab markers, and perhaps slow progression, but few address underlying causes or fully restore health.

Healthcare costs are rising rapidly in the United States, where we are number one in the world in spending, but not in outcomes.

- The U.S. spent $10,345 per person – $3.4 trillion in total – on medical care in 2017. [54]
- Healthcare costs are approaching one out of every five dollars spent in the nation.[55]
- U.S. life expectancy dropped two years in a row in 2015 and 2016 to 78.6 years (and again in 2017), while in 25 other developed countries, life expectancy averaged 81.8 years in 2015, and continues to rise.[56]

Is it possible to unmask the therapeutic illusion without creating major havoc in our society? Although we are number one for spending on medical care, we are not getting our money's worth in return.

Drugs and Medical Devices as a Hidden Health Risk

Another hidden threat is health impacts from prescription drugs and medical devices. Some FDA-approved drugs cause real harm and are pulled off the market after evidence mounts.[57] [58] For others, the FDA lets them stay on the market but issues patient safety communications to alert physicians and patients, and black box warnings of health risks. [59] While some drug impacts reverse when the patient stops the drug, others have lasting health impacts.

The FDA has more stringent regulations for review and approval of prescription drugs than for medical and dental devices, so it is not surprising that installed devices also present "asymmetric threats" to health. They are generally hidden from view inside the body, and not easily considered by physicians and dentists as a source of harm, since they received FDA approval. Applications for FDA approval for devices typically have smaller numbers of patients studied for a shorter time period than prescription drugs.

FDA has more stringent regulations for review and approval of prescription drugs than for medical and dental devices, so it is not surprising that installed devices also present "asymmetric threats" to health. They are generally hidden from view inside the body, and not easily considered by physicians and dentists as a source of harm, as they have received FDA approval.

Applications for FDA approval for devices typically have smaller numbers of patients studied for a shorter time period than prescription drugs. In addition, many devices receive automatic approval because they are "substantially similar" to an existing device – even though they may be made of different materials – and patients' ability to tolerate them varies greatly.[60]

Devices include such materials as nickel, cobalt, mercury (for dental amalgam), other heavy metals, mesh, PET fibers, other plastics, silicone, etc. Patients may have a contact allergy, an autoimmune reaction to device materials, or both, in addition to potential scar tissue and inflammation. Because of the serious impact of these complications and the high cost of device removal and replacement, biocompatibility screening such as a MELISA test and a skin patch test should be done before any device is selected and installed in each patient.

The FDA rarely bans medical devices even after harm is found – only two have been banned in its history.[61] The FDA issues device recalls, patient safety communications, and letters to healthcare providers.[62] However, it often takes many years before enough physicians and patients report harm using the FDA's MedWatch system.[63] It also takes years before they mount a campaign strong enough to get FDA's attention to convene a panel of experts and hold a public hearing, and overcome the opposition mounted by the device company that wants to keep it in unrestricted use.

I tell my patients, if you have an unexplained illness, think dental. Also, think medical devices. AMA can help detect these problems, as they create disturbances in acupuncture meridians. Restoring health can require more than removing the device. It may have caused changes in the immune system, infections, heavy metals or chemicals toxicity, internal damage, and scarring which persist as hidden asymmetric challenges to health.

The Growth of Unexplained or "Mystery Illnesses"

At the same time, we face the growth of unexplained or "mystery illnesses:" chronic fatigue syndrome, fibromyalgia, escalating allergies, autoimmune conditions, autism, cognitive challenges, digestive difficulties, Lyme-associated syndromes, neurological disorders such as Alzheimer's, amyotrophic lateral sclerosis (ALS), multiple sclerosis (MS) and Parkinson's, eczema and skin problems, etc. Each has a constellation of symptoms.

Patients make the rounds from specialist to specialist, each of whom deals with a different system of the body like the blind man feeling the elephant. The treatment to alleviate one problem often does little for the others, and may even create or exacerbate them. Patients either give in or give up, or they begin to seek out alternatives such as complementary or integrative medicine. The practice of functional medicine is also growing, with an expanding set of genomic and laboratory tests. The journey is on. Yet some patients – and medical professionals – are still stymied.

Interestingly, patients' complaints may be the same, that is, they both have fibromyalgia; however from my view, the fibromyalgia is a symptom of underlying problems and not the root problem itself. Therefore, the causes of these symptoms must be determined in order for the patient to achieve their optimum health.

I have seen many patients with chronic fatigue, fibromyalgia, irritable bowel syndrome (IBS), multiple sclerosis (MS), medically unexplained symptoms (which I call MUS), and even cancer patients respond to parasite and antifungal medications and dental revisions.

There are always skeptics who ask, "Have you seen a case like mine? What is your success rate or what is your failure rate?" I have no idea without actually evaluating the patient and may need several visits to see progress. My usual answer is "You are it. There are no statistics to guide or misguide you." Statistics in medicine are not what you call a truly unbiased science when billions of dollars are at stake.

We are internally governed by our beliefs. Whether our beliefs are right or wrong, they still govern our lives and make anything possible or impossible to the person who holds those beliefs. I am not responsible for your cure. You co-create your own healing.

The following articles on extraordinary patients and unexplained diseases illustrate how Acupuncture Meridian Assessment has enabled me to get to the bottom of chronic diseases that have confounded conventional lab tests, gain insights on diagnosis and treatment, and help patients recover their health.

Article: How to Annoy Your Patients and Still Win Them Over: Difficult Doctor on Difficult Patient's DNA Test

On her follow-up visit, Sandy asked me whether she needed to wear a helmet before seeing me. I told her that I was going to wear a helmet myself. I told her that I was hoping that we were wearing helmets on the same team and not against each other.

About 25 years ago, during my early exploration of integrative, complementary medicine, my front desk staff would occasionally ask me, rolling their eyes, what happened to the last patient I saw. He or she had stormed out of the clinic, telling my staff that they will never come back again and that I was rude and did not listen to their problems.

One had severe chronic asthma, brain fog, low back pain, and hip pain. After a thorough evaluation including Acupuncture Meridian Assessment, I told her to see a biological dentist to remove root canals, and to take parasite medications. She found my medical evaluation weird and my recommendations even weirder. How dare I tell her to take parasite medications and to get rid of dental root canals for asthma and body pain when she did not have any GI symptoms or toothache?

These incidents are less frequent now. But, still I will have an occasional confrontational situation in reverse. A patient may fly in from the East or West coast and tell me that he has parasite problems and that nobody can help him. He needs parasite medications for bizarre, crawling sensations on the skin and in the gut. He thinks I am a parasite expert because I've written many articles on the subject.

He went to many infectious disease specialists and parasite specialists from highly regarded medical institutions and either they said that he does not have parasite problems based on a stool test, or they put him on a wimpy dose of parasite medications just to get rid of him. They think he has delusions of parasitosis. He will pull out his smart phone and show me the pictures of parasites in the toilet, or pictures of blood samples taken with darkfield microscopy. Most of them may look like parasites, but they are not parasites. They could be a string of mucous or a fungal formation from a hidden dental infection.

I tell my patients that I am not a parasite specialist, but I treat for parasites based on my Acupuncture Meridian Assessment. I tell my patients that I am sorry, but I cannot justify prescribing parasite medications when their first order of medical care may be seeing a dentist to remove a badly infected asymptomatic tooth. Some of the patients get furious and angry if they do not get parasite medications. They are convinced that they have parasites and I failed to recognize their medical conditions just like every infectious disease specialist. They storm out of the clinic.

It is not my intention to annoy my patients, however if they do not get what they want for their perceived medical care based on an Internet search, they can get hostile and angry. Recently, I saw Sandy, a 72-year-old retired school teacher, from out of town, with main complaints of brain fog, inability to think clearly, bloating, and weight gain. Sandy had seen many medical doctors without much success and was referred by a dentist.

I saw her about 10 years ago and she probably stormed out at that time. This time, she had a DNA test done by her dentist after her tooth extraction and was told by her dentist that she has parasites according to the DNA test and needs to be treated for parasites.

I was annoyed that my patient was telling me how to treat her parasite problems based on her dentist's dental DNA test. I told her that I cannot determine how to treat her for parasites based on a DNA test from the tooth extraction. There are so many variables from the test, and there is no guideline on how to use a dental DNA report to treat parasites. These tests are helpful and can confirm the wisdom of extracting root-canal-treated teeth or oral surgery to clean out jaw cavitations, as you read in my "Battle Plan" for Joe with squamous cell cancer of the thumb in Chapter 6.

When I told her that, she started crying and telling me I am the worst doctor, ignoring the DNA report on parasites. She told me I am the most difficult doctor she has seen in her life. I know we live in a new age of disruptive technology, for better or worse. But, I never heard of a dentist telling the patient to see a medical doctor to treat parasites based on a dental DNA report. It could be a new breakthrough in forensic science for a dental DNA and parasites connection. However, I did not know what to do with this data.

We were locked down, butting heads, and she was crying for two hours in the exam room. Eventually, she calmed down and she told me she can be a difficult patient. We mutually decided that I am a difficult doctor and she is a difficult patient, and we are difficult people. I did put her on a basic detox cleansing program and scheduled a follow up appointment in one month.

On her follow-up visit, she asked me whether she needed to wear a helmet before seeing me. I told her that I was going to wear a helmet myself. I told her that I was hoping that we were wearing helmets on the same team and not against each other. When I told her that, she calmed down.

When I evaluated her with Acupuncture Meridian Assessment, I was able to pick up signals for parasites at the liver, spleen and gallbladder meridians. The indication for the parasite medications, ivermectin, pyrantel pamoate and praziquantel, were quite different than the dental DNA test for parasites. If I followed and treated her based on the dental DNA test for parasites, she may not have responded or may have gotten sicker based on the faulty DNA test, like following fake news.

Her treatment for parasites may take a minimum of three to six months, and requires other nutritional support, a detox program and a monthly gallbladder/liver flush. This time, she was willing to try parasite medications based on Acupuncture Meridian Assessment rather than based on the dental DNA report. We both agreed that I am a difficult doctor and she is a difficult patient. I managed to annoy her but won her back 10 years later, at least for a while.

Article: Do you have MUS? Is This Standard Medical Care by Evidence Based Medicine?

If you've been diagnosed with Medically Unexplained Symptoms (MUS), this article is for you. Evidence Based Medicine is not ready to solve the mystery of MUS.

If you have MUS, Medically Unexplained Symptoms, you are not alone. What are the implications if you have MUS?

A report from the Veterans Administration's (VA) War Related Illness & Injury Study Center of New Jersey, September 2009, explains, "Medically Unexplained Symptoms (MUS) is a term used for health symptoms which remain unexplained after a complete medical evaluation. It's been reported that vague health symptoms account for half of all outpatient visits and that one third of these symptoms remained unexplained after a thorough assessment.

Although common, presence of symptoms which remain unexplained for long periods of time, even after a medical evaluation, can be confusing and frustrating for both patients and providers. Patients who have multiple unexplained symptoms over a period of time may meet the criteria for the diagnosis of the unexplained syndrome (MUS). Being given the diagnosis of MUS can be a relief, although management of these multiple symptoms can be challenging."

I had never heard of MUS as a new diagnosis until I was reading a major medical journal in 2009. I then started searching for the latest information on MUS. The VA report referenced above best summarized and described the concept of multiple unexplainable symptoms. Medically Unexplained Symptoms are often described by people with Chronic Fatigue Syndrome, Fibromyalgia and Irritable Bowel Syndrome. There are many more MUS from unexplainable neurological problems like Autism, ADD/ADHD and Lyme Disease-like symptoms.

If there are so many MUS, how can one treat MUS patients when the "Evidence Based Medicine" taught at medical teaching institutions cannot figure out the cause of the problems? I feel sorry for medical students and doctors in training. Most of MUS patients feel they are out of whack or out of tune, yet, no lab test or medical evaluations shows abnormalities.

After learning the intricate medical science and rituals of clinical training, medical professionals diagnose numerous chronically ill patients as MUS. Medical professionals then end up treating the symptoms with medications for such illnesses as chronic fatigue syndrome, fibromyalgia and irritable bowel syndrome (IBS). This is the current standard medical care! Do you think there's any influence from pharmaceutical companies on our medical training?

I wonder what Galileo Galilee would say about current standard medical care based on Evidence Based Medicine. Galileo, the radical contrarian astronomer of his time, said, "In questions of science, the authority of a thousand is not worth the humble reasoning of a single individual." Most people intuitively understand that something is missing in their medical diagnosis and treatment because they feel something is not right and they know it is not in their head.

Evidence Based Medicine has met MUS! Evidence Based Medicine has been losing credibility and confidence from the public. Evidence Based Medicine is based on measurable and quantifiable science based on linear, compartmentalized thinking which leads to "If everything has to be double-blinded, randomized, and evidenced based, where does that leave new ideas?" (The Lancet, Vol. 366, July 9-15, 2005)

Some of my fibromyalgia patients respond after correcting their dental cavitations (jaw dental infections), IBS patients respond to parasite medications and chronic fatigue patients respond to combinations of dental work, parasite eradications and nutritional therapy. Some of my patients with advanced metastatic cancer respond to intensive detoxification, nutritional therapies and parasite medications and others find that extraction of asymptomatic root canal teeth relieve palpitations, chest pain, arthritic pain and asthma.

So, do you have MUS? Evidence Based Medicine is not ready to solve the mystery of MUS. I propose a new standard medical care that starts with intestinal parasite cleansing, removal of mercury dental amalgams and hidden dental infections, eliminates foods from one's diet that cause food allergies, initiates individualized nutritional programs based on blood or tissue mineral analysis, and includes detoxifications using a gall bladder/liver flush method.

All these combined therapies are a good starting point for most MUS patients. In addition, other tangible and intangible variables may need to be a part of an individualized health plan such as, changes in diet, rest, sleep, stress control, detoxifications and prayer.

Oddly, in the eyes of Evidence Based Medicine, some of the dramatic healing responses to the above regimen are referred to as "placebo effects." Healing often undoubtedly occurs from the above regimen. However, the healing may seem unpredictable and random to an outside observer who doesn't understand this type of healing process since it may not happen instantly and may not occur until a full regimen is utilized over a period of time.

It is sometimes difficult to understand how these individual therapies may or may not be directly related to one's current imminent problems however they are all inter-related. Our body operates according to bio-mechanical, bio-chemical, bio-electrical, and bio-physics means that encompass a unified whole of Body/Mind/Spirit. During the course of these therapies, your body will begin to heal on its own. As you get well, let's call it the "Accidental Cure."

Article: ALS Patient's Unexpected Journey, and Time to Heal at Last: The Story of Ron's ALS

"The ALS Clinic at St. Louis University Hospital, again after even more tests, confirmed the initial diagnosis of ALS. The journey was on. As with the beginning of an unknown journey, there were more questions than answers, more fear than joy, more apprehension than certainty. When the journey involves your very being, another set of emotions kicks in… With the help of my family and friends, I went in search of those people, and I stepped outside of the standard medical world to find answers and to find continued hope…"

> Ronald J. Unterreiner, *An Unexpected Journey: Searching for a cause and finding hope in the battle against ALS*

Several years ago, I wrote an article, "Time to Heal at Last: The Story of Ron's Amyotrophic Lateral Sclerosis (ALS)." I got to know Ron three years ago. He was told by two neurologists that he had ALS based on batteries of neurologic tests in which they were 90 percent sure. He had leg muscle weakness, dragging of his leg, spasms, and his left foot did not always want to cooperate.

The odds were against him to live more than few years after diagnosis of ALS, also known as Lou Gehrig's disease, at the ALS Clinic at St. Louis University Hospital. ALS is one of the most dreaded, progressive neurodegenerative diseases that affect motor neurons. It causes one to lose control of one's muscles, become wheelchair-bound, and eventually, paralyzed and die from respiratory failure.

ALS is a clinical diagnosis made by eliminating all other neurological disorders. When Ron is in a wheelchair and his symptoms become more pronounced, attached to a breathing machine or feeding tube because he cannot swallow, he would be officially diagnosed 100 percent with ALS. He was told by his neurologist that nothing could be done for his ALS and to go home and live as normal a life as possible, and come back every four months to monitor the progression of the ALS. He was not interested in a new experimental drug because of its side effects and limited benefits.

Ron's Book Journey

Ron began to look for alternatives rather than waiting for the inevitable progression of ALS, and he was referred to Prevention and Healing. He said that a wheelchair was not an option for him. He was on a mission, determined, searching for a cause. We embarked on a journey together.

Ron told me he was interested in writing a book to inspire other patients who have ALS. I wrote my article to inspire him to write his book, and he did. Ron's book, *An Unexpected Journey:*

Searching for a cause and finding hope in the battle against ALS, is his personal account of his journey, along with information on the "battle plan" we developed for his treatment.

A recently retired executive in the design and construction industry in St. Louis, Ron stays active in the industry through the nonprofit organization he founded, PEOPLE. It assists minority contractors and helps connect them with majority contractors to more fully participate in the design and construction industry in St. Louis. His book is available for $20 and can be ordered by contacting peopleofconstruction@gmail.com.

I could not put Ron's book down. In addition to giving ALS patients love, peace, and faith in searching for a cause and finding hope in the battle against ALS, the book also speaks to other chronically ill patients on why they need to challenge the medical system. Change your thoughts, change your belief system, change your diet, root out hidden invaders, and change your biological terrain. He describes every step for detoxification to support needed changes in the body. Ron will inspire you with the love, hope, and faith in his writing.

I highly recommend Ron's book not only for patients fighting ALS, but for all chronically ill patients with mysterious illnesses and their families, fellow physicians, and other health-related professionals. This book may save you or your loved one. Ron's book is easy to read, concise, honest, and challenges the current medical system. There are many practical tips and dietary guidelines from his personal experiences.

While I was reading about Ron's journey, I realized that he was teaching me about how to become a better physician. After all, he was describing much of my medical approach to his illness:

searching for the causes. His book also reminded me that I need to take better care of myself.

AMA Assessment and Battle Plan

When Ron first came to me as a patient, Acupuncture Meridian Assessment indicated seven out of 40 meridians were out of balance, including the lymphatic dental point, central nervous system, allergy, heart, liver, and gallbladder meridians.

After the evaluation, I told Ron and his family that I do not treat the diagnosis or symptoms of ALS. I said I would try to remove as much interference (hidden underlying problems) as fast as possible to let the body have time to heal itself. The best I can do is slow down and modify the disease process into a more benign form.

During the course of his treatment, Ron was on antiparasitic medications, antibiotics for dental infections, antifungal medications, and chelation therapy for heavy metal exposures, as heavy metal provocation testing showed moderate amounts of antimony, lead, mercury, and tin.

Ron did numerous courses of insulin potentiation therapy (IPT). His treatment included nutritional supplements and additional detoxification and exercise programs, including crawling daily to reprogram his neural connections and neuromuscular conditioning.

Ron said he previously had 20 plus mercury dental amalgams. Most of them had been replaced, although he had two amalgams left. He also had two root canals at tooth #3 and #18. I told him his amalgams should be removed and the root canals should be extracted as soon as possible by a biological dentist who understands the potential toxic effects of amalgams and root canals.

Ron also had a dental infection at his old wisdom tooth #17. This required an oral surgeon to clean out the infected jaw bone at the site of this tooth. To fix dental-related problems, Ron had two remaining amalgams removed, two root canals extracted, and oral surgery to remove a cavitation in his jawbone at an old wisdom tooth extraction site.

One of the hardest parts of his treatment plan was convincing Ron to have more dental work done, including oral surgery, without any guarantee that the dental work will help him. It took him one year to complete the dental work.

Update

Ron has fully recovered his health and his upper body strength. He is able to do pushups again, when before he needed two hands to lift a cup of coffee or shave. He still has some weakness in his legs and walks with a cane, but has arrested the progression and partially reversed his motor problems. At this stage, my duty as a physician is to monitor and maintain all his meridians in balance, like a well-tuned violin. Hopefully, he has time to heal at last.

In 2017, Ron returned to the neurologist at the ALS clinic who had diagnosed him four years earlier. After reading his latest EMG, the neurologist told Ron that because he had recovered, he "never had it." Perhaps they had made a mistake diagnosing him with ALS a few years ago since all ALS patients have progressive, irreversible neurologic degenerative disease.

I told Ron that he should tap dance when he got better in front of the neurologist to prove that he could reverse ALS and to prove that a "white man can dance." He was a little sheepish about dancing in front of his neurologist, but sent me a picture of him dancing with his granddaughter at a family wedding.

Article: One Hundred Years of Misadventure in Medicine

One of the most overlooked disconnections is the separation of dentistry and medicine as separate and distinct professions. I saw Ayla, a young woman with chronic fatigue, fibromyalgia, and seronegative autoimmune disease. She had seen 29 different medical doctors... Another story tells of my exchange with the U.S. Army European Dental Group Commander, also a full Colonel.

Over the last 100 years there have been major scientific breakthroughs in many medical fields, including the development of antibiotics, surgical mastery of organ transplants, breaking genetic codes, genetic engineering, immunotherapy, stem cells, and anti-aging regenerative medicine. Yet, despite breakthroughs in medicine, there is a strong sense of dissatisfaction.

With all these scientific achievements, these specialized medical breakthroughs are often not interconnected. They often exist without synergies or collaborative efforts across medical fields. They are competing for their territorial fields, as if professional tribal warfare exists between the pharmaceutical industry, hospitals, insurance, and regulatory institutions, such as the Food and Drug Administration (FDA).

One of the most overlooked disconnections is the separation of dentistry and medicine as separate and distinct professions. Recently, I saw Ayla, a young woman with a diagnosis of chronic fatigue, fibromyalgia, and symptoms of seronegative autoimmune disease. She had seen 29 different medical doctors and famous clinics around the U.S. She told me I was the 30th medical doctor she had seen.

In my evaluation, based on a physical exam and Acupuncture Meridian Assessment, Ayla's main problem was coming from an unrecognized dental infection. She could see another 30 different medical doctors, but it would be a fruitless effort to find out what is wrong with her because her medical problem originated from a painless dental infection. Hidden dental infections and unrecognized parasites are often the dominant reasons for patients not responding despite all the "advancements" in medicine.

When I was deployed 10 years ago in Europe in Wurzburg, Germany, at the U.S. Army Combat Support Hospital, I saw a soldier, Frank, with a severe right shoulder pain. He could not raise his arm at all. When deployed for U.S. Army active duty, I would bring my portable equipment to test the acupuncture meridian systems. On my evaluation, his problem was coming from a root canal on his right side. I injected lidocaine at the root canal area and instructed him to move his arm. He was afraid to move his arm because of severe pain. I ordered him to raise his right arm.

To his surprise, within a few minutes, Frank was able to fully raise his arm without any pain. I told him his root canal was causing his shoulder pain. I told him to go to the dental clinic to have the root-canal-treated teeth removed as a long-term solution for his pain. The book, *Root Canal Cover Up*, by George Meinig, DDS, is must reading for all patients (and their dentists) suffering from unexplained medical symptoms.

Two weeks later, I got a very threatening email from the European Commander, a full Colonel for the Dental Group. He was accusatory that I was only a medical Reservist. He said I was meddling with the finest dental group in the U.S. Army and how could I dare to challenge the care of this well-trained dental group. He also forwarded the email to the hospital commander to reprimand my conduct as unprofessional, as a medical doctor challenging dental care.

I was furious at his hostile accusation and demeaning, threatening letter. I emailed him back that the patient did not have a dental problem but a dental-related medical problem. I signed my name with my rank as full Colonel and was hoping this would shut him up. He was using his rank as a full Colonel, Commander of the European Dental Group, to intimidate a medical reservist, and to the hospital commander who is also a full Colonel. I happened to have been promoted to a full Colonel in the U.S. Army before this deployment. I was able stand my ground, rank for rank. If I had been a lower rank, I might have been reprimanded or even punished for recommending the right medical advice.

"Command and control" and "obedience to authority" is a part of the military code. It is the way of operation for military organization. But for real civilian life, it may be considered "bullying." It is time to reexamine the obedience to authority in medical fields by thinking differently.

Game theory is a mathematical model to describe any situation in which the payoffs that participants receive from their actions are at least partly determined by the actions of other people. This could apply to politics, hospitals, selecting your mates for marriage, or selecting your doctors. It sounds very much like quantum effects at the macro level for zero-sum games. The Nobel Prize in economics was awarded numerous times based on Game theory.

Maybe we can come up with a mathematical formula to prove a new odontology: dental, periodontal, neck, and cranium are connected to the rest of the body! It might give us a chance to less selfishly connect and collaborate to solve chronic illness from dementia, neurodegenerative disease, chronic fatigue, fibromyalgia, cancer, heart disease and other mysterious diseases.

Article: Awakening the Healer Within You: Medical Spiritual Wellness from a Bucket of KFC

Sometimes, the best thing for your health is filling your spirit. Read how important a bucket of fried chicken was for one of my patients.

Spiritual Wellness is a part of my lecture series and a part of our prevention and healing program. In the beginning of the lecture, I often ask the audience the metaphysical question, "What if the doctor does not heal and God does not forgive?"

The audience has no problem relating to the idea that the doctor does not heal because they know intuitively that healing must come from within us and not from the doctor. However, I can feel some discomfort from the audience trying to figure out what I am up to by saying "God does not forgive."

At the end of the lecture, I ask the question again, "What if God does not forgive?" I can feel uneasiness and, after a long pause, I ask the audience, "What if God does not forgive because God has nothing to forgive? God embraces all and does not judge, therefore, he does not forgive. Man judges other Men and Men need to learn to forgive others."

I bring this metaphysical question as a way to challenge and hopefully change our thinking. Forgiveness is a very important part of the healing process for any chronically ill patient who does not respond to conventional and other alternative medical care. Often, unresolved emotional conflicts will interfere with our natural ability to heal ourselves. Some of these issues have been addressed in my articles, "Cancer and Cancerous Mind," and "Incurable Disease and Spontaneous Healing."

Fear is the most common negative emotional energy that interferes with our natural healing process. Fear comes in many different energy forms. Fear can transform to self-doubt, jealousy, suspicion, anger, or blame. It will interfere at every level of the spiritual, mental, emotional, and physical body; all causing physical manifestations.

Fear is highly profitable for many businesses. When there was a murder in my neighborhood, I got constant sales phone calls from home security system companies promoting their products in the name of security. Pharmaceutical companies promote and sell drugs with sleek advertisements highlighting various fears: fear of cancer, heart attack, cholesterol, erectile dysfunction, or suffering of a loved one.

The financial, insurance and legal systems thrive on selling fear, for which the cure is financial security or legal justice. For politics and religion, I better keep my mouth shut. After all, the End of America and Armageddon are the biggest, most profitable ways to promote fear for profit for right or wrong reasons.

Every day, I face patients with many unexplainable medical symptoms. They are given medical diagnoses with many creative Latin names which only add more anxieties and fear. They may have advanced metastatic cancer, been warned of an imminent heart attack from severe blockage of the coronary artery, or have an "incurable" autoimmune disease with a whole list of physical sufferings.

Their medical diagnosis becomes their identity: "I am a breast or prostate cancer patient," "I am a cancer survivor," "I am a Lyme or chronic fatigue and immune dysfunction syndrome (CFIDS) patient," etc. When you correct the five common underlying problems – hidden parasites, food allergies, nutritional deficiencies, dental problems, and detoxification including chelation therapy for heavy metal toxicity – often the problem resolves on its own. You may call it spontaneous healing, placebo effect or "accidental cure."

Joan, a 67-year-old nurse with ovarian cancer, first diagnosed in 2006, came to see me in February 2010. She had a total hysterectomy and chemotherapy, but she had recurrent metastatic cancer with a rapidly rising cancer marker, CA-125. Thirty-two out of 40 acupuncture meridians were out of balance on her first visit.

Joan was started on intestinal detoxification, parasite cleansing, dental work, heavy metal chelation therapy, and nutritional support including high dose IV vitamin C. She was anemic and required blood transfusions. Overall, she appeared relatively stable, at least not rapidly deteriorating with current therapy. However, her CA-125 continued to rise, and she decided to do chemotherapy although she did not believe in chemotherapy.

During the course of the treatment, I noticed she had a peculiar fear about food and was losing weight. She had so many reasons why she could not eat, although she had very few food allergies and had a good appetite. One day, she told me she was craving chicken strips but was afraid to eat.

To make the story short, I told Joan I was not sure how she would respond to my therapy, but it was okay for her to eat her chicken without any fear regardless of the outcome. I told her on her way home to stop by and get a bucket of KFC and eat with her family and enjoy every piece of chicken.

I have not seen Joan since her last visit, but I was told she did stop by at Piccadilly cafeteria and picked up a bag of her favorite chicken strips to share with her family. I am not sure a bucket of KFC or chicken strips will help her cancer at the physical level, but eating her favorite chicken without fear, and overcoming that fear, will nourish her mind, emotion and spirit.

Jim, a 55-year-old man with a history of heart attack, came to see me recently. I told him he did not have a heart attack because he was eating steak. His cardiologist forbade him to eat steak for the last several years. I told him he had a heart attack from hidden dental problems and told him to get his favorite T-bone steak and enjoy every bite of it. He promised he would see the dentist and have his infected root canals removed. You should have seen his eyes, in disbelief, fill with joy and tears.

Many patients like Joan or Jim need extra-dimensional efforts to promote healing, which I like to call Medical Spiritual Healing. Overcoming fear, whether it is a bucket of KFC or T-bone steak, is one of the most important first steps to understand the awakening of the healer within you.

Part 5
Parasite Medication Guidelines for Physicians

Chapter 12 Parasite Medication Guidelines: for Physicians, Medical Hackers and Braves

I learned that using parasite medications was the fastest way to rebalance all the meridians, except the dental-related and allergy/immunology points.

This chapter, written for physicians, gives background on the decision-making process for choosing parasite medications, a set of Parasite Medication Charts (organized by medication and by parasite), and guidelines for taking parasite medications. It may also be helpful for patients who want a deeper dive into the topic.

Decision-Making Process for Choosing Medications: Bolivia and U.S. Army Connection

Physicians and patients always ask me how I started using parasite medications extensively in my practice. My response is based on a combination of U.S. Army field medicine and how those experiences informed my clinical practice in the United States.

During a Medical Corps field deployment with the U.S. Army in Bolivia in 2001, we administered thousands of rounds of parasite medications to thousands of people in a two-week period. They reported not only resolution of first-line parasite problems, but improvements in many other chronic health problems.

This had a profound impact on me: parasites could cause chronic inflammation and result in a host of medical problems not typically seen as related. Treating an underlying problem resulted in healing seemingly unrelated chronic conditions and diseases. I called this phenomenon, "accidental cure," and my experiences became the basis of my first book, *Accidental Cure*.

In my clinical practice in the United States, I began to explore the potential that parasite problems underlie a range of chronic health problems in patients who did not respond to conventional care. The challenge was that stool and blood tests for parasites were often negative. I learned that parasites are masters of deception, and can go to great lengths to avoid detection to ensure their survival.

I began to integrate more systematic use of parasite medications in my clinical practice when unexplained symptoms persisted that were suggestive of parasite problems, and when problems on relevant meridians were indicated by Acupuncture Meridian Assessment (AMA) testing. Patients began to report spontaneous resolution of many modern chronic illness including asthma, autism, cancer, IBS/IBD, and persistent Lyme.

Before our mission to Bolivia in 2001, I was already familiar with Acupuncture Meridian Assessment – I was trained in EAV by Dr. Doug Cook, DDS and many others. I used herbal parasite remedies recommended by Hulda Clark, PhD, ND, such as wormwood, black walnut hull, and clove oil with good success for common intestinal problems. I wrote articles on her work on my website.

After this mission, I began using pyrantel pamoate and/or mebendazole – the medications we dispensed at the U.S. Army medical team in Bolivia. I noticed not only my patients describing that their intestinal problems were resolved, but also their asthma, bronchiectasis, chronic fatigue syndrome, fibromyalgia, MS brain lesions resolved, and even cancerous conditions stabilized, as described in my book, *Accidental Cure*.

Because I could not prove that they actually had parasites by Western standard medical evaluation, I could not claim that the patients had parasites. If they got better, I called it an "accidental cure," since claiming without proof is considered unscientific or even fraud in the eyes of medical boards and the academic community.

Choosing Parasite Medications

Many physicians have asked for more information on how, why and what dosages to use for the certain conditions. This chapter is my best effort to explain the most frequently asked questions about choosing medications based on Acupuncture Meridian Assessment (AMA), a modified version of Electro-Acupuncture according to Dr. Voll (EAV). EAV uses principles of homeopathy, is cumbersome to learn, and takes too much time to assess. By default, I developed AMA to fit into my need as an internist with a military background, to get to the point, and use the KISS (keep it simple, stupid) principle.

I learned that using parasite medications was the fastest way to rebalance all the meridians, except the dental-related and allergy/immunology points. Allergy/immunology points are associated with not only food and airborne allergies, but also heavy metal exposure, fungal/mycotoxins, and environmental toxins, including glyphosates, residual Agent Orange, petrochemicals, and insecticides.

Four Major Categories of Parasites

There are four major categories of parasites: protozoa, roundworms (nematodes), tapeworms (cestodes) and flukes (trematodes). Each responds to different types of medications. Some patients report a new kind of parasite, "rope worms." Forget them – they are most likely a type of biofilm from an accumulation of mucus in the intestinal tract. Rope worms are considered the equivalent of Russian Fake News or a Russian hoax by parasitologists.

Introduction to Parasite Medications

Since 2001, I have tried many different combinations of medications to rebalance the meridians. These medications are what I use over 80% of the time on my patients, based on AMA assessment. Despite what you might read on the Internet, I do not have a protocol – but these should be considered my favorite parasite medications.

These are the most common medications I use all the time. I will use many different combinations, as described later in this section. Once, I used five different parasite medications at the same time on a physician. He was afraid the massive parasite medications would kill him, but in fact, he got better.

Most Common Parasite Medications I Use

Here is a list of the most common parasite medications I use, with typical dosages and duration (for 150-180 lb. person):

Ivermectin 12mg 3-4 x/day with **pyrantel pamoate** 725 mg 3-4 x/day for 10-30 days

Tinidazole 2000 mg at bedtime or 500 mg 3-4 x/day, up to 30 days, or **nitazoxanide (Alinia)** 500 mg 2-3 x/day for 3-10 days

Albendazole 200-400 mg 4 x/day for skin problems or **mebendazole** 100-200 mg 4 x/day for 2-4 weeks

Praziquantel 600 mg 4 x/day for 2-4 weeks

Matching Medications to Meridian Imbalances

Each imbalance in a meridian seems to respond better to certain types of parasite medications. Based on 18 years of clinical experience since the Bolivia mission and my four-day training courses on AMA and parasite medications for physicians, here are the corresponding meridians and parasite medications:

- Large (LI) and Small (SI) Intestine meridians: ivermectin, pyrantel pamoate, albendazole, mebendazole. Note: If diarrhea is present with LI or SI imbalance, add tinidazole or Alinia
- Gallbladder/Liver/Spleen/Pancreas meridians: praziquantel
- Stomach/Spleen meridians: tinidazole, doxycycline, Zithromax
- Triple Warmer meridian on Breast: tinidazole and treat dental infection
- Kidney meridian: heavy metals, dental, parasites
- Bladder/Uterus/Prostate meridians: tinidazole, praziquantel, ivermectin
- Cancer: all of the above, plus antifungal meds

Medications Used for Indicated Parasitic Conditions

Table 2 provides a list of parasite medications and indicated parasitic conditions, according to the medical literature. Table 3 follows with a summary of medications listed by parasite.

Parasite Medication Charts – By Medication

Table 2. Parasite Medication Chart - By Medication

Ivermectin

Treatment	<ul><li>Filariasis: Onchocerca volvulus (river blindness) for onchocerciasis. Take additional dosage at 3, 6, 9 and 12 month intervals</li><li>Cutaneous larva migrans of dog and cat whipworm</li><li>Strongyloidiasis (threadworm, a roundworm)</li><li>Trichuriasis (whipworm)</li><li>Head or pubic lice and scabies</li></ul>
Notes	<ul><li>May combine with pyrantel pamoate and praziquantel</li><li>Contraindicated in children under 5, and those breastfeeding, and with hepatic or renal disease</li></ul>
Pharmacology	<ul><li>Broad-spectrum antiparasitic agent</li><li>Derived from bacterium, Streptomyces avermitilis</li><li>Binds and activates glutamate-gated chloride channels: invertebrate-specific members of the Cys-loop family of ligand-gated ion channels present in neurons and myocytes</li><li>Does not cross the blood-brain barrier of mammals (except tortoises) due to presence of P-glycoprotein</li></ul>

Pyrantel Pamoate

Treatment	<ul><li>Hookworms of all species</li><li>Roundworms like Ascaris</li><li>Pinworm</li></ul>
Notes	<ul><li>May combine with praziquantel for tapeworm</li></ul>

	• May combine with febantel for whipworm • May induce intestinal obstruction in a heavy worm load from trying to pass a large number of dislodged worms at once
Pharmacology	• Acts as a depolarizing neuromuscular blocking agent, thereby causing sudden contraction and paralysis of helminths. This causes worms to lose grip on the intestinal wall and be expelled by natural processes

Nitazoxanide (Alinia)

Treatment	• First line treatment for protozoa Cryptosporidium parvum and Giardia lamblia • Also indicated for chronic hepatitis B and C and influenza virus A
Notes	• Discovered in the 1980s by Jean-Francois Rossignol at Pasteur Institute
Pharmacology	• Works due to interference with pyruvate ferredoxin oxidoreductase (PFOR) dependent electron transfer reaction which is essential to anaerobic energy metabolism

Tinidazole

Treatment	• Amoebic protozoal infections • Trichomoniasis • Giardiasis • Amoebiasis
Notes	• Common side effects include upset stomach, bitter taste, itchiness and disulfiram-like reactions with alcohol such as nausea, vomiting, headache, flushing and shortness of breath

Pharmacology	• Chemically similar to metronidazole with similar side effects • Developed in 1972

Praziquantel (Biltricide)

Treatment	• Schistosoma fluke • Fasciolopsis buski, intestinal fluke • Chinese liver fluke, Clonorchis sinensis • Some tapeworms, hydatid disease and larval stages of Echinococcus • Cysticercosis caused by infection of brain or muscles with eggs and larvae of the pork tapeworm, Taenia solium • Toxocariasis • Paragonimus westermani, lung fluke • Diplozoon paradoxum and other Trematoda infections from eating sushi
Pharmacology	• The mode of action is not exactly known, but it increases the permeability of the membrane of schistosome cells toward calcium ions. It induces contraction of the parasites, resulting in paralysis in the contracted state. • Praziquantel interferes with adenosine uptake in cultured worms.

Mebendazole (Vermox)

Treatment	• Roundworm • Hookworm • Pinworm • Whipworm • Other worms
Pharmacology	• Selectively inhibits the synthesis of microtubules in parasitic worms and destroys extant cytoplasmic microtubules in their intestinal cells,

	<ul><li>thereby blocking the uptake of glucose and other nutrients, resulting in the gradual immobilization and eventual death of the helminths.</li><li>Oncologic treatment potential with significantly inhibited cancer cell growth, migration and metastatic formation of adrenocortical carcinoma, both in vivo and in vitro.</li><li>Mebendazole induces a dose- and time-dependent apoptotic response in human cancer cell lines, and apoptosis via Bcl-2 protein inactivation in chemotherapy-resistant melanoma cells.</li></ul>

Albendazole (Albenza)

Treatment	<ul><li>Roundworms</li><li>Tapeworms</li><li>Flatworms: Flukes/Trematodes, Tapeworm/cestodes, Echinococcosis</li><li>Nematodes: Hookworms</li><li>Whipworms</li><li>Pinworms or threadworms</li><li>Cutaneous larva migrans</li><li>Toxocariasis</li></ul>
Notes	<ul><li>Combine with ivermectin or diethylcarbamazine</li><li>Hydatid Disease: 400 mg 2x/day for 28 days on 14 days off for 3 cycles</li><li>Neurocysticercosis: 400 mg 2x/day for 8-30 days</li><li>Filaria: 400 mg single dose</li></ul>
Pharmacology	<ul><li>Albendazole causes degenerative alterations in the intestinal cells of the worms by binding to the colchicine-sensitive site of tubulin, thus inhibiting its polymerization or assembly into microtubules.</li></ul>

	• The loss of the cytoplasmic microtubules leads to impaired uptake of glucose by the larval and adult stages of the susceptible parasites, and depletes their glycogen stores. • Degenerative changes occur in the endoplasmic reticulum, the mitochondria of the germinal layer, and the subsequent release of lysosomes.

Metronidazole (Flagyl)

Treatment	• Antibacterial, amoebicidal and antiprotozoal • Anaerobic bacteria, Clostridium difficile • Bacterial vaginosis of Gardnerella + anaerobes • Pelvic inflammatory disease • Anaerobic bacteria with abdominal abscess, peritonitis, empyema, pneumonia, lung abscess, diabetic foot ulcer, meningitis, brain abscess, bone and joint infection, tubo-ovarian abscess or endocarditis • Pseudomembranous colitis due to Clostridium difficile • Helicobacter pylori • Amoebiasis, Giardiasis, Trichomonas vaginalis • Acute gingivitis and other dental infections
Notes	• When combined with mebendazole, higher risk for Stevens-Johnson syndrome • For Crohn's, combine with Cipro
Pharmacology	• Metronidazole is reduced to disrupt energy metabolism of anaerobes by hindering the replication, transcription and repair process of DNA, resulting

	in cell death. The presence of oxygen prevents reduction of metronidazole and hence reduces its cytotoxicity.

Iodoquinol/Diiodohydroxyquinoline (Yodoxin)

Treatment	• Amoebiasis: Entamoeba histolytica, active against cysts and trophozoites
Notes	• Poorly absorbed from the GI tract and is used as a luminal amoebicide
Pharmacology	• Acts by chelation of ferrous ions for metabolism. The full mechanism of action is unknown.

Niclosamide

Treatment	• Treats tapeworms; praziquantel used more frequently due to side effects • Treats Schistosomas • Shows promise as anti-cancer agent for colon, prostate, kidney, breast and other cancers
Notes	• Anthelmintic activity • Potential antineoplastic (anticancer) activity, three clinical trials underway
Pharmacology	• Inhibits glucose uptake, oxidative phosphorylation, and anaerobic metabolism in the tapeworm • *In vivo* & *in vitro* activity against methicillin-resistant Staphylococcus aureus (MRSA) • Inhibits proliferation of colorectal cancer cells and has little to no toxicity toward nonmalignant tissues • Induces apoptosis of cancer cells in both prostate and breast cancer cell lines.

Parasite Medication Charts – By Parasite

Table 3. Parasite Medication Chart - By Parasite

Amoebiasis (Entamoeba histolytica)	• Iodoquinol 650 mg po tid for 20 days • Metronidazole • Tinidazole • Paromomycin
Amoebic Meningoencephalitis	• Amphotericin B 1.5 mg/kg/day IV in 2 doses x 3 days, then 1.0 mg/kg/day for 6 days plus intrathecally 2x/day, then 1.0 mg/day every other day for 8 days
Ancylostoma (Eosinophilic enterocolitis): Hookworm	• Albendazole • Mebendazole • Pyrantel pamoate
Ascariasis	• Albendazole • Mebendazole • Ivermectin
Babesiosis	• Clindamycin plus quinine 650 mg po tid 10 days • Atovaquone 750 mg bid 10 days,+ • Azithromycin 600 mg qid 10 days
Balantidiasis (Balantidium coli)	• Tetracycline 500 mg qid 10 days • Metronidazole 750 mg tid 5 days • Iodoquinol 650 mg tid 20 days
Cryptosporidiosis (Cryptosporidium)	• Nitazoxanide (Alinia) 500 mg bid 30 days
Cutaneous Larva Migrans (Hookworm)	• Albendazole • Ivermectin
Enterobius (Pinworm)	• Mebendazole for 2 weeks • Pyrantel pamoate for 2 weeks • Albendazole for 2 weeks

Flukes:	
Clonorchis sinensis (Chinese Liver Fluke)	• Praziquantel 75 mg/kg/day in 3 doses • Albendazole 10 mg/kg/day
Fasciola hepatica (Sheep Liver Fluke)	• Praziquantel • Albendazole • Nitazoxanide
Fasciolopsis buski (Intestinal Fluke)	• Praziquantel • Albendazole • Nitazoxanide
Paragonimus westermani (Lung Fluke)	• Praziquantel • Albendazole • Nitazoxanide
Giardiasis	• Metronidazole 250 mg tid 7 days • Tinidazole 2000 mg once • Nitazoxanide 500mg bid 3 days
Gnathostomiasis	• Albendazole • Ivermectin • Surgical removal
Gongylonemiasis	• Albendazole • Surgical removal
Hookworm (Ancylostoma duodenale, Necator americanus)	• Albendazole • Mebendazole • Pyrantel pamoate
Isosporiasis (Cystoisospora belli)	• Trimethoprim/sulfamethoxazole DS (Bactrim DS) bid for 10 days
Leishmania (Visceral and Cutaneous)	• Amphotericin B • Sodium stibogluconate • Miltefosine • Paromomycin IM 15 mg/kg/day IM 21 days
Lice	• Malathion .5% • Permethrin 1% • Ivermectin

Loa Loa (Filariasis)	• Diethylcarbamazine 6 mg/kg/day in 3 doses for 12 days, plus antihistamines and/or steroids to decrease the allergic reaction • Tropical Pulmonary Eosinophilia – diethylcarbamazine • Onchocerca volvulus (river blindness) – ivermectin
Malaria	• Quinine sulfate 650 mg tid 7-10 days, plus doxycycline 100 mg bid, or plus tetracycline 250 mg qid, or plus clindamycin, or • Atovaquone/proguanil, or • Artemether/lumefantrine or • Mepacrine/quinacrine, or • Mefloquine, or • Quinidine gluconate
Microsporidiosis (ocular, intestinal or disseminated)	• Albendazole
Pneumocystis jirovecii (carinii)	• Trimethoprim/sulfamethoxazole • Primaquine plus clindamycin • Dapsone plus pyrimethamine or Pentamidine • Atovaquone
Schistosomiasis (Bilharziasis)	• Praziquantel 40 mg/kg/day in 2 doses 1 day
Strongyloidiasis	• Ivermectin • Albendazole
Tapeworms:	•
Fish (Diphyllobothrium latum)	• Praziquantel
Beef (Taenia saginata)	• Praziquantel • Niclosamide
Pork (Taenia solium)	• Praziquantel • Niclosamide
Dwarf Tapeworm (Hymenolepis nana)	• Praziquantel • Nitazoxanide

Echinococcus granulosus (hydatid cyst)	• Albendazole 400 mg bid for 1-6 mos
Toxoplasmosis	• Pyrimethamine 25-100 mg/day for 3-4 wks plus sulfadiazine 1-1.5 g qid 3-4 wks
Trichomoniasis	• Metronidazole • Tinidazole
Trichinellosis	• Albendazole or mebendazole plus steroids for symptom control
Trichostrongylus	• Pyrantel pamoate • Mebendazole • Albendazole
Trichuriasis (Whipworm)	• Mebendazole • Albendazole • Ivermectin
Trypanosomiasis T. cruzi (American trypanosomiasis, Chagas)	• Nifurtimox 8-10 mg/kg/day in 3-4 dose or benznidazole
Trypanosomiasis T. brucei gambiense (West African Trypanosomiasis, Sleeping Sickness)	• Pentamidine or suramin, eflornithine or melarsoprol
Visceral Larva Migrans (Toxocariasis)	• Albendazole • Mebendazole

Parasite Remedies: Guidelines for Taking Medications

Here are the guidelines for taking parasite medications I share with my patients:

You have been advised to take parasite medication(s) and you might be wondering, "Yuk! Do I really have worms in my body? Dr. Yu didn't even check my stool. How does he know what kind of parasites I have? How does he know how to treat them?"

Most parasites are invisible, microscopic, and outside of the intestinal tract. I recommend you go to my website at www.preventionandhealing.com. Look at the "Articles" page for articles on parasites, and for the ones titled "Accidental Cure" and "Luthiers and Physicians." Also read all of the Testimonials and Success Stories pages. That may seem like a lot of reading. You just have to ask yourself, "Is my health worth taking the time to really understand what's going on with me and why I should take this medicine?"

Most patients tolerate the medications well and will complete the round of medications. Some patients have a strong reaction depending on the medications. Reactions can also result from the effects of killing the parasites. Reactions may include nausea, fatigue, dizziness, rashes, itching, abdominal cramps, or diarrhea. Don't be alarmed. These symptoms are only temporary. If you cannot tolerate the medications, stop them and contact the office for advice.

Most of the time, you will be instructed to stop the medications for 48 hours. Then resume at half the dose and finish the medications. Rarely, you will be instructed to stop the medications altogether.

You may take over-the-counter medications, such as Benadryl or Pepto-Bismol, to relieve some symptoms of itching or upset stomach. For whatever reason, if you cannot tolerate the medications, stop and call the clinic the following working day.

Every person's situation needs to be addressed for their particular condition. It is not uncommon, though, that parasites can move from one organ to another and transform into different patterns of impact on your body. For this reason, it is sometimes necessary to use different types of parasite remedies at different times over a period of time.

For example, sometimes different remedies are used in a specific sequence. At other times, one remedy may be used for a while, and your condition may indicate the absence of parasites only to have them return some months later. At this second occurrence, a different remedy may be required. Each situation is unique and will be treated only according to what your body is telling us.

Wish you all the best on your journey of recovery and wellness.

Background Explanations Addressing Common Questions

We have been programmed to believe that parasites infect people who live in tropical countries like Africa, Mexico, India and China, but not the United States. You may be warned about parasites only if you travel to those countries. You may have been told, "If you don't travel outside the U.S. you don't have to be concerned about parasites."

However, for the last 50 years there has been a large global migration of people into the U.S. In addition, global warming is creating an unprecedented opportunity for new emerging infectious diseases including parasites. On top of this is environmental pollution that has been destroying our ecosystems. This may provide a friendlier environment in which parasites can flourish.

Parasites have been associated with every known disease in the history of humankind. I consider parasites one of the five principal causes of a large percentage of all illnesses. The others are: heavy metal toxicities, hidden dental problems, food allergies, and nutritional problems.

Herbal parasite remedies are generally not strong enough to kill deeply embedded parasites in the body. I will often add prescription parasite medications and homeopathic intestinal remedies to have the maximum killing effect. Most parasites have a very complex lifecycle outside of the intestinal tract and require a relatively high dose and multiple treatments.

For patients without access to prescription medications, updated information on herbal approaches to treating parasites is available from Steven Buhner, *Healing Lyme*, and the Parasitology Center website of Omar Amin, PhD, www.parasitetesting.com. Some of my patients have tried the Rife frequency generator. The Rife frequency generator does not penetrate deeply enough into organs like the liver or gallbladder. It may be partially effective at best.

One of the most frequent questions I encounter is, "Is my parasite infestation contagious to my family members?" It all depends on the parasites and how you acquired them. Not everybody will catch parasites from contaminated water or foods. It depends on your immune system, the strength of your stomach's ability to produce hydrochloric acid, and your body's ability to destroy parasite eggs embedded in foods.

However, if you have recurrent parasite-related problems while being very careful with your dietary intake, I may recommend your spouse and other family members living with you be evaluated by a doctor familiar with parasite infestation. I also recommend having your pets checked for parasites by your veterinarian. (I don't test your pets. I draw the line.)

Patient Consent Form for Parasite Medication Usage Disclaimer

In my practice, I have a five-page consent form for patients outlining background to help patients decide whether they wish to receive treatment involving parasite medications, the use of parasite medications, therapies involved and other treatment options, and potential risks and benefits. The patient agrees that they have read and understand the information, no assurances or guarantees were made, they have been fully informed about the treatment procedure, possible benefits, and risks associated with parasite medications, provided a full patient history, and will promptly inform staff if they experience side effects or discomfort. The consent form is designed to minimize or eliminate liability based on full disclosure. The patient must sign the disclaimer before they get the prescribed medication.

Article: Healing Crisis by Herxheimer Reaction: Is This Side Effects or Lazarus Effects?

Here is an article on the Herxheimer Reaction (also known as "healing crisis") that I share with my patients.

Old country medical doctors often talked about the "healing crisis," the cleansing reaction after they administered herbs or medications. They would often be at the bedside monitoring their patient going through extreme fever, chills, nausea, diarrhea, cramps, and skin eruptions with boils, hives or rashes, and with a strong emotional release or even delusions.

So, what is the healing crisis? It is also known as the Herxheimer Reaction. This reaction occurs when the body tries to eliminate toxins at a faster rate than the body can properly dispose of them. The most common reaction occurs as bacteria or yeast dies off during the course of antibiotics or antifungal medication. Although less well known, antiparasitic medications can also trigger Herxheimer reactions, but most physicians do not have enough experience with these medications.

Adolf Jarisch, an Austrian dermatologist, and Karl Herxheimer, a German dermatologist, are credited with the discovery of the Jarisch-Herxheimer or simply Herxheimer reaction. The reaction was first seen following treatment in early and later stages of syphilis treated with mercury or antibiotics. It is seen in 50% of patients with primary syphilis and 90% of patients with secondary syphilis.

Why is it important for you to understand the healing crisis, the Herxheimer reaction? It is a lot more common than you think. However, most people assume the reaction is side effects of the medications and not a part of the healing process. As a consequence, they stop the medications out of fear.

The more you are chronically ill with the burden of toxins in your system, the more severe the detoxification reaction or healing crisis you may experience. It is characterized by a temporary increase in symptoms during the cleansing or detox process.

But these reactions are instead signs that the treatment is working and that your body is going through the process of cleansing itself of the toxins. Such reactions are temporary and can occur immediately or within a few days after starting the medical treatment. Symptoms usually last a few days and rarely last for weeks. Often, what you experience during the healing crisis may be identical to the disease itself.

What can you do when you experience the healing crisis or Herxheimer Reaction? Drink plenty of filtered water to keep your body well hydrated and to flush the toxins. You may also use herbal tea or vegetable juice and start a coffee enema or colonics to assist the detoxification by increasing the rate at which your body can rid itself of the toxins. If you are still feeling fatigued or sleepy, be kind to yourself, rest during the day and get plenty of sleep at night.

If you are not responding to the above steps, call your doctor. You may need to reduce the dosage or temporarily stop the medication under your doctor's supervision. The Healing Crisis is part of the healing process and not necessarily the side effects of the treatment or medications. Knowing the difference between the healing crisis and the side effects of the treatment is not so obvious. That is considered the Art of Medicine.

One of my patients described her journey of the healing process in her testimonial, titled, "You Have Given Me My Life Back," on my website, www.preventionandhealing.com. It took her several years to recover from the effects of mercury poisoning and the neurological symptoms she was experiencing. Her treatments included chelation therapy, dental work, nutritional support, and detoxification. She described her experience of recovery as the "Lazarus" in her. Her full description of her healing process is described in my book, *Accidental Cure*, in chapter 17, "Lazarus Effects." When the healing crisis has passed, you may feel as though you too experienced the Lazarus Effect.

Frequently Asked Questions for Using Parasite Medications

Question: Which parasite medications should I use?

Answer: Based on Acupuncture Meridian Assessment and the corresponding disturbance of each meridian.

Question: What is the dosage and duration of treatment?

Answer: I started with the PDR-guided dose and realized that for chronically sick patients, they needed much higher doses in different combinations, and going through several cycles. Treatment can last 6-12 months.

Question: Which combinations of parasite medications to use?

Answer: See above lists, and the section earlier in this chapter, "Most Common Parasite Medications I Use." The specific combinations are based on acupuncture meridian assessment, clinical review and my experience, and will vary among patients.

Question: Which medications balance which specific meridians?

Answer: See above lists, and the section earlier in this chapter, "Matching Medications to Meridian Imbalances." The specific medications are based on acupuncture meridian assessment, clinical review and my experience, and will vary among patients.

Question: Do you use a compounding pharmacy?

Answer: Because you may need to adapt dosages of some of the medications, you may find it helpful to use a compounding pharmacy. At times, this can also result in savings for the patient, as the prices of some standard generic drugs have skyrocketed.

Question: Do you combine prescription antiparasitics with herbal and homeopathic remedies?

Answer: I may still use herbal parasite remedies, such as Hulda Clark's classic wormwood, black walnut hull and clove oil, to cover the entire basis. However, they are not strong enough to treat established infections.

Question: When is the best time to start the medications?

Answer: Prepare patients before starting medications; otherwise they may have an intense healing crisis, called a Herxheimer reaction. See my article, "Healing Crisis by Herxheimer Reaction," earlier in this chapter. The bowels must move daily before starting parasite medications. Support the organs with liver, kidney, lymph, allergy and drainage support based on homotoxicology principles.

Question: Do you treat using the moon cycle or a different life cycle for treatment?

Answer: Once patients complete the first long multiple-parasite-medications phase and survive their baptism with parasite medications, switch to short maintenance cycles during full moon cycles for 6-12 months. If people do not respond, I may use a new moon cycle and tweak and change the combination of medications.

Question: What kind of side effects or side benefits are there?

Answer: Refer to the article, "Healing Crisis by Herxheimer Reaction," located earlier in this chapter.

Question: What about prescribing medications without a confirmed diagnosis?

Answer: This is the most challenging part from the physician's point of view. We were trained as a scientist and clinician to get proof of parasite infestations before prescribing meds, creating a mental block for physicians. Go slowly and gain more experience using medications by training on how to use AMA training with me, or learn to use Autonomic Response Testing (ART) developed by Dietrich Klinghardt, MD, PhD, from Germany.

Question: How do you handle patients who are suspicious and in doubt?

Answer: Start with natural and homeopathic remedies before trying prescribed parasite medications. These patients will often go back to their physicians to verify if they really have parasite problems, and stool test for ova and parasites are usually negative. Their physicians will dismiss your findings, so accept that most of these patients will not come back.

Question: What do you do when EAV/AMA reading is normal but you are still suspicious of parasites?

Answer: When partially treated with natural or prescribed medications, all meridians may appear balanced and normal, yet problems persist. It requires advanced training to uncover hidden problems. I have nicknamed this, "Operation Open Sesame" or "Enhanced Interrogation Technique" (OOPS or EIT). This hands-on technique is beyond the scope of this book to describe without attending the AMA training. There are a variety of techniques to unmask and reveal these problems, which otherwise confound physicians and patients alike. You need to be open minded for quantum entanglement/quantum effects and embrace a 5,000-year-old disruptive new technology.

Another approach is to do a short therapeutic trial of parasite medications, to see if it is effective.

For more background on my unusual, nonstandard, high-dose combination approach to parasite medications, see my article, "Big Whack Theory," in Chapter 7 on Parasites. To recap: "Higher doses of combinations of parasite medications often give fewer side effects than using lower doses or fewer medications. The U.S. Army Combat Casualty Care Course (C4) dictates that, 'Superior fire power is the best preventive medicine.' If you use a lower dose of parasite medications, you might be engaged in a Whack-a-mole game of never-ending hide and seek."

*   *   *

For physicians seeking more information on detecting and treating parasite problems (as well as dental and fungal problems), you may consider attending one of my AMA Training Sessions, which are offered twice yearly in St. Louis, Missouri.

Part 6
For Patients

Chapter 13 For Patients: Self-Help Strategies and Resources

Most of the recommendations are free or inexpensive (under $100)
except dental care.

The following articles outline actions you can take to help safeguard and improve your health:

- One Hundred Dollar Cure for Braves, Skeptics and El Cheapo
- Ten Dollar Cure When One Hundred Dollar Cure Fails
- Gallbladder-Liver Flush
- Folk Remedy from Russia: Oil Therapy by Dr. Karach
- Detox Recommendations Based on Great Plains Lab Test Results
- Self-Help Resources on the Web
- How to Find a Biological Dentist
- Maximus and Minimus: Cure for All, Cure for None

First, here is a story to share with you:

A woman brought a very limp duck to see a veterinary surgeon. As she laid her pet on the table, the vet pulled out his stethoscope and listened to the bird's chest. After a silent moment, the vet shook his head and sadly said, "I am sorry, your duck is dead." The women protested, "How can you be so sure? You haven't done any testing on him. He might just be in a coma or something else." The vet rolled his eyes, turned around and left the room.

He returned with a black Labrador retriever. The dog sniffed the duck from the top to bottom, and the dog looked up at the vet with sad eyes and shook his head. The vet patted the dog on the head and took it out of the room. A few minutes later, he returned with a cat. The cat jumped on the table and also delicately sniffed the bird from head to foot. The cat shook his head, meowed softly and strolled out of the room.

The vet looked at the woman and said, "I am sorry, but as I said, this is most definitely, 100% certifiably, a dead duck." The vet turned to his computer terminal, hit a few keys and produced a bill, which he handed to the woman. The duck's owner, still in shock, took the bill. "$150 just to tell me my duck is dead!!!" The vet shrugged, "I am sorry. If you had just taken my word for it, the bill would have been $20, but with the Lab Report and the CAT scan, it's now $150."

One Hundred Dollar Cure for Braves, Skeptics and El Cheapo

Most of my patients come to see me for a second opinion after traditional therapies have failed. They may have chronic fatigue, fibromyalgia, irritable bowel syndrome or more serious problems with ulcerative colitis, unexplainable chest pain, or cancer.

Most of them no longer have confidence in our current medical system, and they are interested in taking care of themselves. They are a self-educated new generation of contemporary, brave, and self-reliant frontier men and women surfing the Internet as their primary source of alternative medical information.

One of the hardest parts of practicing integrative medicine has been that it is not recognized by insurance companies. They will not pay for my evaluation based on Acupuncture Meridian Assessment and recommended integrative therapies.

The biggest barrier from seeking medical advice in my practice has been financial considerations, since I do not accept insurance. Actually, it is the other way around. The medical insurance does not accept my medical practice because I practice non-standard complementary medicine.

Because finance is the limiting factor, I educate my patients on self-help and simple steps to regain their health. Sometimes a patient asks me if I can cure their complicated medical problems for $100. This article provides many simple tips for those who are interested in taking care of themselves and with limited financial resources who need a practical solution for a myriad of medical symptoms.

- Start your day with raw eggs, milk, butter and nuts/nut butter.
- You must drink more water with sea salt and no soda, diet soda or juice.
- Regular bowel movement (1-3x/day). You may use ground flax seeds, intestinal herbal cleansing or extra natural fibers from fresh vegetables.
- Oil pulling therapy recommended by Dr. Karach for all chronic medical conditions (later in this chapter).
- Gallbladder/liver flush four times per year (see instructions later in this chapter).
- Get a suntan for free vitamin D or take 2000 to 5000 units of vitamin D 3x/day.
- Take high-potency multivitamins and minerals with extra vitamin C 1000-3000 mg/day.
- Limit your coffee, and your whiskey, to less than 2-3 cups or shots or equivalent beverages/day.
- Take extra iodine or kelp.
- Follow the Enter the Zone diet by Dr. Barry Sears and the Eat Right for Your Type blood type diet by Dr. Peter D'Adamo.

- Take apple cider vinegar with meals and add honey when you feel exhausted.
- Try Dr. Coca's <u>Pulse test</u> for an elimination diet and save money on a food allergy diet (his book is on Amazon).
- Think of geopathic disturbance and electromagnetic field interference as a cause of illness.
- When you are in doubt, avoid all grains, processed dairy products and soy or soy milk.
- When you are still in doubt and not feeling well, eat liver, honey and take cod liver oil.
- Deworm twice a year. Black walnut hull, wormwood and cloves are classic Native American herbs.
- Avoid those people who drain your energy. Avoid energy vampires.
- Daily five rites yoga stretching exercises (see article on my website, Holistic Exercise Program and the "Five Rites").
- Dental Death Trap: If you have dental-related unexplained medical problems, this is the most expensive part of your medical care. Look for a good biological dentist.

If you still have multiple unexplained symptoms (MUS), it is time to see a holistic, integrative medical doctor.

Ten Dollar Cure When One Hundred Dollar Cure Fails

After I wrote, "One Hundred Dollar Cure: Cure for Braves, Skeptics and El Cheapo," one of the readers wrote a letter stating he is not an "El Cheapo." He is simply broke and wants medical advice for $10.

Below is a more detailed list of recommendations on how to save money and take care of yourself, your family members and loved ones with $10 cures.

1) Stop cholesterol-lowering statin drugs. It will save you a lot of money. Instead, take niacin 500 mg 3 times per day for a few cents per day. Ignore your cholesterol level and eat three to six raw or slightly cooked organic eggs per day. You may read my article on my website: "Cholesterol Therapy Based on Compromised Science: My Apology for Telling You the Truth."

2) Stop anti-acid medications like Prevacid, Zantac or the latest purple pills. Try digestive enzymes and apple cider vinegar for a few cents per day. You will be surprised – most of your heartburn and digestive problems will disappear, and you will feel better. Recommended reading of my articles: "Acid Reflux and Rebellious Stomach: Killing the Messenger for Profit," and "Apple Cider Vinegar, Forgotten Ancient Remedy: A Holy Grail for Fountain of Youth."

3) Give up wheat and corn and your wheat belly and corn butt will disappear. Most pig farmers know how to fatten pigs: feed them corn. Our government recommends a low-fat diet and an increase in whole-grain complex carbohydrates. At the same time, Americans are suffering from wheat belly and corn butt. Dr. William Davis, MD, a cardiologist, recently published a book, *Wheat Belly: Lose the Wheat, Lose the Weight, and Find Your Path Back to Health,* in which he extensively covers the scientific basis for the folly of modern wheat and gluten sensitivity. It is a must-read. Go to the library. It is free and it may save your life. If you have diabetes, high blood pressure, fatigue, body aches, irritability, or brain fog, try a no-wheat and no-grain diet for at least three months. Also, make sure you eat lots of green and colorful vegetables. A doctor's visit may not be necessary.

4) Try the oil pulling therapy recommended by Dr. Karach. It is good for all chronic medical conditions. Swish one tablespoon of sesame oil, peanut oil or sunflower oil for 20 minutes, spit it out,

and then brush with baking soda and salt. For more information, see my article, "Folk Remedy from Russia," later in this chapter.

5) Try Five Rites and yoga exercise daily. Long-distance running is not recommended unless you are addicted to running. Brisk walking or hiking is much easier than running on your feet, knees and hips. Exercise is free! Recommend reading my article, "Holistic Exercise Program and the 'Five Rites.'"

6) For sleeplessness and insomnia. Sleep is important for your health and beauty. Remove all electronic devices, including TV, phones, and radios in the bedroom, and sleep in total darkness. You may add melatonin, GABA, L-hydroxytryptophan and L-theanine. Doses are dependent on individuals. Resolve any conflicts for the day through mediation, open communications, meditation or prayer before going to bed.

7) Deworm twice a year with Native American herbs like black walnut hull, wormwood and cloves. You may need prescription parasite medications. For example, a horse's average life span has doubled from routine dental care and deworming 2-4 times per year. Ask your veterinarian. Anti-aging therapy may start with routine deworming and oil pulling for dental/oral hygiene. Consider these options before thinking of hormone replacement therapy.

8) Gallbladder/liver flushes every season. Think of this as the body's need for an oil filter change every 3 months. You can find the instructions later in this chapter.

9) Get a suntan. Sunlight is free but do not get sunburned. Do not use sunblock lotion. Take vitamin D3 2000 to 5000 U/day. When you catch colds or flu, double or triple the dose for 10 days.

10) When in doubt, eat liver, take more iodine, and spend more time with your loved ones. Avoid people who will make you feel more tired, depressed or drained. Drink more water and less beer or whiskey.

11) Keep cheerful friends and companions. Surround yourself with the things you love: family, pets, music, plants or nature. Get away from dead-end relationships and dead-end jobs. Enjoy simple things. In the long run, we are all dead. Laugh and let go of fear, anger and guilt.

12) Pray. It is okay to pray and ask help from the higher being. Science only deals with the relative truth. Spirituality deals with the truth. "God is dead, said Nietzsche; Nietzsche is dead, said God."

Additional Therapies to Consider

Those with additional resources may want to consider some additional therapies to assist with detoxification and oxygenation.

These help to rebuild your body and cells, restore your gut, and reboot your mind, metabolism and pathways. They include:

- Pulsed Electromagnetic Frequency (PEMF)
- Exercise with Oxygen Therapy (EWOT)
- Vibration Platform
- Infrared sauna

Acupuncture, chiropractic, wellness counseling, meditation, therapeutic massage, and other healing modalities provide a foundation for recovery and vitality. As part of an initial consultation, patients can choose a visit with an acupuncturist or a wellness counselor located in my practice.

Detox Recommendations Based on Great Plains Lab Test Results

Based on the patient's Great Plains Lab Results, we may consider the following recommendations to assist detoxification. These are general recommendations, not a protocol.

Additional Testing if not done or if indicated:

- Hair mineral analysis and recommended supplements, food allergy sensitivity testing and recommendations.
- DMPS heavy metal challenge test, mycotoxins, organic acids test, hormone profile, etc.

Helpful Activities

- High-fat diet, food allergies rotation diet, blood type diet, read *The Plant Paradox* for caution regarding lectins.
- Sweat therapy of any kind, exercise, sun exposure.
- Infrared sauna.
- Coffee enema daily and colonics once a week based on the individual.
- Gallbladder/liver flush monthly or quarterly for 12 months.
- Bentonite clay, mud pack, mud bath.
- Sleep: no electronics in the bedroom, consider melatonin, GABA, L-hydroxytryptophan, L-theanine, etc.
- Limit exposure to electromagnetic frequency (EMF), cell phone, radio frequencies, microwaves, wireless, and radon.
- Circuit training: Pulsed Electromagnetic Frequency (PEMF), Exercise with Oxygen Therapy (EWOT), Vibration Platform, and Infrared Sauna.

Intravenous (IV) Therapies

- IV vitamin C, and/or combination of IV and UV/ozone.
- IV Patricia Kane (PK) protocol plus liposomal glutathione and phosphatidylcholine, such as BodyBio PC.

Supplements (as directed)

- Colon and whole body cleansing.
- Kidney, Liver, Allergy, and Lymph Drainage support.
- Charcoal 1 capsule 3 times per day between meals and meds.
- Probiotics and prebiotics nutritional support: Green Drink.
- Increase oral vitamin C, E, lipoic acid, glutathione, N-Acetyl cysteine (NAC).
- Hormonal support.
- Emotional stress control: 5-HTP, L-Tryptophan, homeopathic supports, and/or Bach flower remedies.
- Nutritional support with vitamins and minerals.
- Homeopathics, such as Chem Tox, Neuro Tox, Pesticide Tox, Lymph Drainage.

Gallbladder/Liver Flush Instructions

I recommend my patients do a <u>Gallbladder/Liver Flush</u> four times a year. The instructions below are also given on my website, which you may check for updates from time to time.

Drink plenty of filtered water containing no chlorine or fluoride. On average, drink 8 glasses of water, 8 oz. each, per day between meals. Do not drink water with your meals because it dilutes your gastric juices and may cause indigestion and malabsorption.

Cleansing Your Colon and Your Body

The gallbladder/liver flush is a quick, easy and inexpensive way to cleanse the liver, the most important organ system for detoxification, or "detox."

How to do the Gallbladder/Liver Flush (see Figure 22 at end):

STEP 1:

Add 8 droppers of Ultra-Phos Liquid in one quart of apple juice and mix well. (One "full" dropper usually only fills about half of the physical length of the dropper.) Drink at least 1 quart of high-quality apple juice daily for 3 to 4 days. If you have diabetes or sensitivity to sugar, you may substitute a mixture of up to 1 part apple juice with 1 part filtered water; add 8 "full" droppers of Ultra-Phos Liquid per quart. Take malic acid plus magnesium, 500mg 1 tab a day. This will help thin your bile and make it easier to pass from your liver and gallbladder. Eat light meals.

STEP 2:

On the 3rd or 4th day of Step 1, do the following: 2-3 hours prior to drinking olive oil, take 1 teaspoon to 1 tablespoon Epsom salt in 12 oz. of water. Drink 1/2 cup of extra virgin olive oil. For taste, you may mix it with 1 cup of cola beverage and the juice of a whole fresh lemon (room temperature). You may also use the juice of a whole grapefruit. Drink this mixture in the evening or at bedtime on an empty stomach (at least 4 hours after the last meal). Try not to drink the mixed oil all at once but within 15-30 minutes.

Dinner should be a light and low-fat meal. Those with diabetes can use a diet cola beverage. If you have gone through this flush without any response, for the next flush you can increase the amount of olive oil up to 1 cup or as tolerated. *The cola beverage is an option and NOT required.*

STEP 3:

Immediately after you drink the olive oil, lie down on your right side with your knees up to your chest for at least 30 minutes. The oil stimulates the liver and gallbladder to purge the sludge bile and get it to flow. Next day, after your bowel movements, you will probably see many green objects. They usually start to come out after the 2nd or 3rd bowel movement. Some people may pass green objects for several days.

Occasionally you may need an herbal laxative to get things moving or several large warm water enemas or colonics. *If you experience any abdominal discomfort or cramps, take 1 additional tablespoon of Epsom salt in a 12 oz. glass of water.*

Questions and Answers

Question: Do you feel pain with the gallbladder/liver flush?

<u>Answer</u>: No, however, you may feel nauseated for a few hours. The cola beverage and lemon juice will help to settle your stomach. You may use grapefruit juice instead of lemon juice.

Question: Do I have to follow these exact instructions?

<u>Answer</u>: No, there are many various methods of gallbladder/liver flush programs. You may do a daily flush with a smaller dose of olive oil, or try different types of oil such as grape seed oil or flax seed oil, if olive oil is not tolerated or available.

Question: How long and how often do I have to do this program?

Answer: We recommend once every other week until passing very few stones, then monthly. Gradually taper to 4 times a year (for every season) for maintenance.

Question: If my gallbladder has been removed, can I still do the gallbladder/liver flush?

Answer: Yes. You will need more than ever to get rid of the sludge of bile and toxins from the liver.

Question: Is there any danger in doing the gallbladder/liver flush?

Answer: It is possible for gallstones to get stuck in the bile duct, where they may cause acute inflammation of the gallbladder. However, if you use apple juice and Ultra-Phos Liquid you shouldn't have any problems. We have never seen a complication as long as you follow all the instructions carefully.

Question: Are the green objects real stones?

Answer: The initial bowl passage may contain true gallstones. However, most of the green objects are congealed bile sludge mixed with olive oil coming out of the liver and gallbladder ducts. They still have toxins, and parasites can lay their eggs in them, so it is best to get rid of it. The goal is to kill and purge parasites.

Question: Do I still have to take all my other medication while I'm taking the gallbladder/liver flush?

Answer: Olive oil may upset your stomach so we recommend not taking any medication, vitamins or minerals for 6 hours before and 6 hours after taking olive oil.

Question: Is this the only detox program I need?

Answer: Perhaps not. This is a simple basic detox program. If you are very toxic, you may need an advanced individualized intense detox program, including high enemas or colonics.

Question: If I don't pass any green objects should I stop the program?

Answer: Some people may have to do more than 2 or 3 gallbladder/liver flushes before they start passing green objects. About 60-70% of people will notice green stones on the first trial.

Figure 22. Gallbladder/Liver Flush Timeline

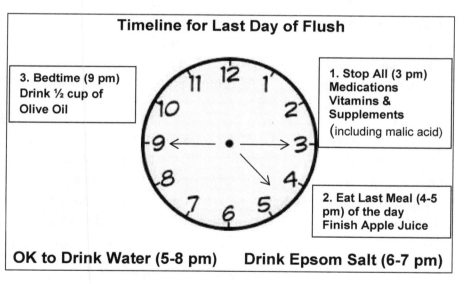

Folk Remedy from Russia: Oil Therapy by Dr. Karach

Folk remedies have an endearing quality for mankind because they are simple, easy to use and often effective. The most well-known folk remedies are garlic and apple cider vinegar. In Russia, garlic is considered to be a Russian antibiotic comparable to penicillin in America.

The other well-known folk remedy is apple cider vinegar, which I described in a previous article. Chicken soup for colds and duct tape for warts are other well-known folk remedies. What about oil therapy? This is not some exotic aromatic oil but what you can buy from your local grocery store.

This lesser known folk remedy of oil therapy from Russia was introduced by Dr. Karach., MD. He presented a paper to the All-Ukrainian Association of the Academy of Science of the USSR. He explained an unusual simple healing process using cold-pressed oils.

The exciting feature of this oil therapy is its simplicity. It consists of swishing cold-pressed vegetable oil in the mouth. The healing process is accomplished by extracting toxic waste without disturbing the healthy microflora. Dr. Karach says humans are living only half of their potential life span. They could potentially live to be 140 to 150 years old by simply following his oil therapy.

Dr. Karach claims the oil therapy is effective for the following conditions: headache, bronchitis, lung and liver conditions, toothache, thrombosis, blood disorders, arthritis, paralysis, eczema, gastric ulcers, intestinal disorders, heart and kidney conditions, encephalitis, nervous conditions, and other disorders.

The best oil to use is cold-pressed sunflower seed oil or natural peanut oil. If you have a hard time getting cold-pressed oil, you can use regular sunflower oil or peanut oil. In the morning before breakfast on an empty stomach, take 1 tablespoon in the mouth but **do not swallow it**. The oil is slowly swished in the mouth and drawn through the teeth for 15 to 20 minutes.

It is thoroughly swished in the mouth and drawn through, chewed and mixed with saliva. Chewing activates the enzymes and the enzymes draw toxins out of the blood. **The oil must not be swallowed because it becomes toxic.** The oil gets thinner and white. It is then spit from the mouth into the sink or toilet.

If the oil is still yellow, it has not been masticated thoroughly or long enough. After the oil has been removed from the mouth, rinse with warm water mixed with a 1/2 teaspoon of sea salt and baking soda several times. Then, brush gums, teeth and tongue with salt and baking soda. If you have chronic sinusitis, you may also gently sniff up the mixed salt and baking soda water to clean the nasal and sinus passages.

If Dr. Karach is correct, this simple oil therapy is preventive as well as curative. He states, "With the use of this therapy, I healed my chronic blood disease of fifteen years. I was healed within three days of an acute arthritis that forced me to lie in bed."

I believe Dr. Karach's oil therapy is a simple and elegant way to solve common dental-related medical problems. This oil therapy is an excellent dental hygiene self-care therapy. Your visits to your dentist and medical doctor will be less frequent. After all, I never enjoyed going to the dentist. For that matter, it's even worse to be evaluated by a medical doctor. I recommend that all my patients follow his regimen. Thank you, Dr. Karach! This is a gift of love from Russia.

Self-Help Resources on the Web

People increasingly find health information on the Web and share experiences on social media. In addition to conventional medical sites, there are many web-based sites and webinars on integrative and complementary medicine, biological dentistry, and more. Patients share experiences in Facebook groups and chat groups for a wide variety of health problems.

Susan L., PhD, one of my patients who is an MIT engineer and whose family had escalating health problems, developed a fascinating website based on what she learned in hacking her family's parasite and related health problems, Debug Your Health, www.debugyourhealth.com. In it, she covers 18 topics they dealt with, sharing helpful information and resources. My article on her experience, "Parasite Treatment Hacked by an MIT Engineer: Think Small, Dream Big for Pandemic," is included in Chapter 7.

Another website is Better Health Guy, www.betterhealthguy.com, written by Scott Forsgren, whose stories are included in this book. He suffered very serious chronic illnesses, and was diagnosed with mononucleosis, chronic Epstein-Barr virus (EBV), chronic fatigue syndrome (CFS/CFIDS), fibromyalgia (FMS), severe food allergies, leaky gut syndrome, parasitic infections, multiple sclerosis (MS), heavy metal toxicity, Candida, Western equine encephalomyelitis (from a mosquito bite), Lyme disease, Ehrlichia, Bartonella, Babesia, HHV-6, and others. His website contains a blog, podcasts and more.

How to Find a Biological Dentist

Because it is so important, I am including this information here, as well as in Chapter 6 on Dental.

There are three associations of biological and holistic dentists in the United States, which also have international members. Each provides a listing of members on its website. Here is their contact information.

International Academy of Oral Medicine and Toxicology (IAOMT)
8297 ChampionsGate Blvd, #193 ChampionsGate, FL 33896
(863) 420-6373
Website: www.iaomt.org
Find a dentist: https://iaomt.org/for-patients/search/

International Academy of Biological Dentistry and Medicine (IABDM)
19122 Camellia Bend Circle Spring, Texas 77379
(281) 651-1745
Website: www.iabdm.org
Find a dentist: https://iabdm.org/location/

Holistic Dental Association
1825 Ponce de Leon Blvd. #148 Coral Gables, FL 33134
(305) 356-7338
Website: www.holisticdental.org
Find a dentist: http://holisticdental.org/find-a-holistic-dentist/

Article: Maximus and Minimus: Cure for All, Cure for None

In my practice, I see many chronically ill patients who have been seen by many medical doctors and are often considered incurable. They were told to learn to live with their medical conditions, how medications will ease their suffering and help to manage the progression of disease... Your medical problems may not be what you think, what you have been told, or diagnosed. It is up to you...

I was in Paris for my honeymoon as a young physician. I studied French for three years in high school and thought it would be good to test my recall of the language. The hotel was very modest. Our typical daily activities included walking to one museum after another.

One evening, I noticed a restaurant named Maxim's, the famous restaurant I heard about in the movies where famous people like to have dinner and hang out. I suggested to my newly wedded wife, Kate, we go to Maxim's for dinner. When we entered the restaurant, I was not impressed. It looked clean and nice but not as special as I expected. The crowds looked very ordinary and the food was fine but nothing special.

My experience at Maxim's was a big disappointment compared to my great expectation. In my imagination, Hemingway and Humphrey Bogart were smoking cigars, drinking cognac, eating fine French cuisine and surrounded by beautiful French women. However, the place was half empty, no music, and we didn't see any extraordinarily beautiful French women.

As we left, I looked up at the restaurant and told myself, "Maxim's is totally overrated. I would never recommend it to anyone." However, to my dismay, when I saw the sign for the restaurant, it said "Minim's." I was so sure the sign said Maxim's when I entered the restaurant. I don't think I can blame this on my rusty French.

Why am I bringing up the story of Maxim's and Minim's? It is our unrealistic expectations that distort our perceptions of reality. Minim's was a fine restaurant, but my expectation was unrealistic for Minim's to fulfill my imagination of Maxim's.

I think our medical system often creates unrealistic expectations, in the same way that my expectation of Maxim's became my experience with Minim's, as we purportedly provide the best medical care in the world. This is especially true when we are dealing with chronic illness.

I've written numerous articles that discuss how many medical problems are not true medical problems, but are "problems" created and marketed to give an illusion that you are sick. This continuously growing trend is promulgated by multinational pharmaceutical companies who often promote their drugs in the name of awareness of "early screening" and "public education" for every conceivable medical condition. For more information, look at my article, "Cure for All Diseases and Non-Diseases: Let's Start with Honey Bee Erectile Dysfunction."

If you have certain medical conditions like high cholesterol, acid reflux, mild hypertension, menopausal symptoms, arthritic pain, fibromyalgia, osteopenia, erectile dysfunction, attention deficient, or memory problems, advertisements gently remind you to ask your doctor about specific drugs, in a slick TV commercial, to promote medications that are based on pseudoscience and the psychology of fear.

Most people understand that when they have a life-threatening medical problem like an acute heart attack, pneumonia, asthma, trauma or cancer, they have no choice except acute medical intervention to stop the immediate medical conditions with maximum effort. After all, Western medicine excels in crisis management and trauma care. However, emergency care is very different than treating chronic illness. Western medicine can excel in one area but not the other.

In my practice, I see many chronically ill patients who have been seen by many medical doctors and often considered incurable. They were often told to learn to live with their medical conditions and how their medications will ease their suffering and help to manage the progression of the disease.

To make my story short, your medical problems may not be what you think, what you have been told, or what has been diagnosed. I do not treat individual symptoms based on a single diagnosis. I evaluate the whole body based on Acupuncture Meridian Assessment, the modern biocybernetic matrix system, which gives me an informational clue where to start. Depending on the circumstances, most people need to start with intestinal cleansing, parasite eradication, heavy metal detoxification, nutritional support, elimination of food allergies, and/or correcting hidden dental problems by seeing a biological dentist.

During the course of the evaluation and treatment, patients often observe a "spontaneous healing" or, as I like to call it, "accidental cure." At times, though, I don't see much response from my therapies. It happens more often when patients have unrealistic expectations or are skeptical and only willing to try part of my recommendations. For them, it can be a disappointing experience.

You can create your own success or failure for your incurable medical condition. It is up to you. Learn how to create the opportunity for "spontaneous healing." Your healing experience could be like Maxim's or Minim's or I should say, "Maximus and Minimus: Cure for All, Cure for None."

Conclusion

> *What if the "accidental cure" concept catches on, is taught, shared, recreated and multiplies? It may manifest in the AcciDental Blow Up in Medicine!*

Is it possible to reconstruct new medicine based on new biology using the ancient wisdom of Acupuncture Meridian Assessment (AMA)? Is there a role for Energy Medicine and restoring a healthy biological terrain in caring for cancer, Lyme, and mysterious chronic illnesses? Is it possible to blend integrative and complementary medicine with the current bifurcated medical-dental model? I hope this book gives you compelling reasons why we must bridge the gap between Western and Eastern medicine, and fully integrate medical and dental care, along with other natural healing programs.

If you need more motivation to embark on a journey and develop a battle plan for health as a patient – or as a physician – or as a dentist – these examples may provide some additional support.

U.S. Army Vet, 67, with Lymphoma

Bob, a 67-year-old U.S. Army Vietnam veteran came to see me about seven years ago with aggressive B-cell lymphoma. He refused chemotherapy recommended by the VA hospital. I did my usual treatment based on Acupuncture Meridian Assessment to correct the underlying dental, parasites, fungal, and heavy metal problems, along with referrals for dental work needed, and detoxification strategies outlined in this book.

I was able to slow down the progression of his lymphoma, but he still had severe ulcerating lymphoma under his left armpit. I told him that I did the best I could, and asked him to try chemotherapy which he had refused to do previously.

When I recommend chemotherapy, most of my patients think I am giving up on them, and they do not return. I told him we did a lot of cleansing, detox and reducing his infectious burden, and if somebody would respond to chemotherapy it would be him. As a side comment, I added that he may not need the full dose of chemotherapy; who knows, he may need only half the recommended dose. That was our last conversation.

Six years passed and I did not see him. He never came back for a follow-up visit, and I thought he had died from a complication of lymphoma and chemotherapy. To my surprise, one year ago, he came back, with a very unusual request. He had received a letter one week before from the VA, denying his 100% disability and saying he now had zero disability. He no longer had lymphoma and was considered cured.

He asked me for some kind of statement to write to the VA hospital on why he still needed disability benefits. I reviewed his chart and all his labs were fine except for slightly abnormal kidney function, probably from chemotherapy. His ulcerated lymphoma was completely healed on physical exam, and there was no evidence of lymphoma on CT scans.

I told him I had not seen him for six years and I thought he had died, and I asked him what he did. He said he did as I told him and decided to do chemotherapy. He decided to stop on his own after half the recommended course, as his ulcerating lymphoma had healed. His lymphoma never came back.

Maybe, he was lucky. In addition, all the dental work, parasite medications, detox, cleansing and nutritional support might have helped him make that happen. I told him he needed to take his wife out for dinner to celebrate! He had beaten lymphoma without any major side effects. It was time to celebrate, not seek disability. He can get a job at Walmart if he needs to. Celebrate first. Get a job later.

Sharon, Professor, with Persistent Lyme

Remember Sharon, the 60-year-old college professor from upstate New York? Sharon is a classic Lyme patient who provides a forensic case study. Here is a quick recap of her story.

Sharon had a tick bite in 2013 and was on doxycycline and initially felt better. A year later, she was told she had seronegative Lyme disease. Two years later, she experienced vision loss with white clouding on her vision, but the eye exam was normal. Since then, she experienced right eye pain and pins-and-needles- like pain. She has seen 13 physicians, and none of them knew what was wrong.

A spinal tap in January 2017 was positive for Borrelia. She was officially diagnosed with CNS neurologic Lyme disease. An infectious disease specialist started her on a 28-day course of IV ceftriaxone, and there was no improvement. She was told her Lyme disease was treated, and she now has Lyme syndrome. She experienced persistent tingling arms and legs, incontinence, lower back pain, fibromyalgia pain all over, severe fatigue, loss of appetite, weight loss, and severe insomnia.

Sharon went to a Lyme clinic in Arizona. There, she received a 10-week course of IV antibiotics and six weeks of insulin potentiation therapy (IPT). Unfortunately, she developed pancreatitis during the course of treatment. Next, she had oral surgery in Colorado for four cavitations and replacement of two amalgams. She also had a coffee enema, during which she passed "two different kinds of parasites" – the admissible evidence – and came to see me for parasite problems.

Acupuncture Meridian Assessment (AMA) showed that 8 out of 40 meridians were out of balance. Her gallbladder, allergy/immunology and small intestine meridians were the dominant problems. She was started on parasite meds: ivermectin, pyrantel pamoate, and praziquantel; followed by antifungal meds: fluconazole and itraconazole; and other support therapies.

On her second visit, she reported feeling much better, and all her 40 meridians were balanced. She will be on multiple rounds of alternating parasite/antifungal meds. This is a long process of eliminating several layers of infections – including Borrelia burgdorferi and co-infections – with IV antibiotics, dental cavitation (jawbone) infections with oral surgery, and finally, parasites and fungal infections with potent prescribed medications.

It may be premature for me to say she is healing from persistent Lyme. Time will tell. From the forensic science of who committed the crime, her missing links between Lyme disease and persistent Lyme syndrome were her dental infections (four jawbone cavitations) and parasite/fungal infections.

Construction Contractor, 58, with Parkinson's Disease

I saw Bill, a 58-year-old construction contractor with newly diagnosed Parkinson's disease, who was on medication to control his tremors and stiffness. His dominant problems were coming from the dental and allergy/immunology points based on Acupuncture Meridian Assessment (AMA), with a high index of suspicion for environmental toxins. His urine test for toxic chemicals showed extremely high petrochemical based toxic chemicals: MTBE, ethylene oxide, bromopropane, and propylene oxide. While he was diagnosed with Parkinson's disease based on his symptoms, the cause of his tremors was from toxic chemicals.

I routinely check for heavy metals like lead, mercury, cadmium, aluminum, nickel, tin, and tungsten, and treat these patients with chelation therapy, nutritional support and a general cleansing program. Many people respond to the program, but some of the sickest people do not respond until you also get the environmental toxic chemicals out.

A Tale of Two Physicians

About four years ago, I saw two physicians with the same diagnosis of chronic lymphocytic leukemia (CLL), one from Florida alligator country and one from La La Land. I focus on uncovering underlying problems, not on their diagnosis. Most of the treatment plans are similar. Get rid of parasites and fungal problems, correct any dental problems, check for heavy metals and start chelation therapy based on which toxic metals are the dominant problems. Put patients on nutritional support based on hair mineral analysis, food allergy testing and Blood Type diet. Dealing with dental-related medical problems is the most difficult area to convince my patients to take action.

These two physicians were open to integrative/complementary medicine and highly motivated to follow my recommendations and instructions. The physician from La La Land responded like a classic La La Land story; not only did his leukemia resolve – his severe psoriasis, diabetes and hypertension also resolved. I have not seen him for the last several years, but he says all is fine. It is hard to convince a busy physician to come back for a routine follow-up checkup.

On the other hand, to my disappointment, the physician from Florida did not respond to my therapies. His blood counts were fluctuating, but kept going up. He thought pulsed electromagnetic field (PEMF) therapy made the situation worse by stimulating his bone marrow, and stopped PEMF. But his blood counts continued to rise despite intense nutritional and IV therapies, and reached a critical level of over 600,000 white blood cells (WBC). The normal range is 3,400 to 10,800 WBC.

He had emergency plasmapheresis by a hematologist in Florida. He took an experimental, expensive drug, ibrutinib, per his oncologist, and stopped coming to see me for almost two years. His blood count dropped to normal at 8,000 WBC, and he stopped the ibrutinib because of the side effects. His WBC counts started rising again, and he came back to see me for reassessment of his condition.

Because he did not respond to my usual and customary treatment plan, I decide to test for environmental toxic chemicals based on Acupuncture Meridian Assessment (AMA). Surprisingly – or perhaps not – he had massive amounts of petrochemical-based toxic chemicals including MTBE/ETBE, diethyl phthalate, styrene, benzene, perchlorate, diphenyl phosphate, and bromopropane, and organophosphate insecticides, according to Great Plains Labs. He was also exposed to high levels of the herbicide glyphosate and fungal toxin ochratoxin A, considered a carcinogenic mycotoxin.

Now I understand why he did not respond to my usual treatments. His blood counts were going in the wrong direction. He also had heavy metals including mercury, parasites and fungal problems. It will take him months or years to detoxify his toxic burden.

For common environmental toxic chemical exposures, a home detox program includes a gallbladder/liver flush once per month, coffee enemas, sauna or sweat therapy, charcoal or bentonite clay, mudpack, and vitamins and minerals.

These environmental chemical toxins and heavy metals are silent killers that our medical professionals overlook, as they typically treat the symptoms based on an arbitrary diagnosis. The other silent killers are parasites, fungal/mycotoxins and hidden dental-related medical problems.

The mystery of the tale of these two leukemia patients was separated by environmental toxic chemicals. By the way, I found out on his last visit that the Florida doctor was not doing the gallbladder/liver flush which is a part of all my cancer patients' detox program. In fact, he had never done the gallbladder/liver flush during the last four years, as he did not want to drink apple juice because of his concern for fruit sugar content. The mystery of the Florida alligator doctor was not as mysterious as I thought. It seems like miracle stories only come from La La Land.

Time to Work Together

These are good examples of why we need to work together as doctors, dentists and patients in developing battle plans to fight underlying causes of diseases and restore health. Whether you have cancer, Lyme, or mysterious chronic illness, if all else fails, it is time to explore hidden parasites, dental problems, fungal mycotoxins, environmental chemicals, heavy metals, detoxification, and nutritional support.

As I noted in the Preface, this is especially important, given all the challenges we face today: 1) hidden invaders: parasites, mold/mycotoxins, viruses, bacteria, and other infections; 2) the environment: heavy metals, toxins and pollutants; 3) what we ingest: food and beverage products, food additives and GMOs; 4) pharmaceuticals and medical/dental devices that can cause side effects as well as benefits; 5) accidents and physical and emotional trauma; and 6) sedentary lifestyles in a wirelessly connected digital world and widely interconnected physical world.

Today, our medical system is designed more for the benefit of "stakeholders" and shareholders than patients. Instead of investors asking if curing patients is a sustainable business model, we should be asking: How can we help patients get better? The disconnection between paying for costly drugs and lifelong medication management – but not for prevention and integrative therapies – is striking. Patients suffer as doctors and dentists diagnose and treat the human body as separate organs to be cared for by specialists, instead of looking at it holistically as an integrated, subtle energetic symphony of systems.

What if the "accidental cure" and asymmetric threat concepts catch on, are taught, shared, recreated and multiply? It may manifest in the AcciDental Blow Up in Medicine.

Prevention and Healing is the way to bring health, people, family and community together. As integrative physicians and holistic, biological dentists, together we can help patients overcome cancer, Lyme, and mysterious chronic diseases. We can retire the standard current medical/dental practice model, and help patients on a journey, armed with a battle plan against asymmetric threats. This is your battle plan for life!

About the Author

Dr. Simon Yu, MD

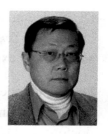

Dr. Simon Yu combines internal medicine with integrative medicine at Prevention and Healing, Inc., which he founded in 1996. Dr. Yu received his B.S. degree from Washington University, and did postgraduate research in diabetes at Washington University Medical Center. He earned a Master of Science degree through a joint program at Washington University Medical Center and University of Missouri-St. Louis, where he conducted research on immunology. He graduated from the School of Medicine at the University of Missouri in 1984 and completed residency training at St. Mary's Health Center in St. Louis.

Dr. Yu worked as a regional medical director at a large health maintenance organization (HMO) medical group in Missouri for 10 years. He also served as a medical officer in the U.S. Army Reserve for 25 years, further expanding his experience. Dr. Yu experienced first-hand the limits of Western medicine's and HMO health systems' medication-management approach to patients with cancer and chronic diseases. He began studying integrative and complementary medicine over two decades ago. He took 300 hours of acupuncture training at Stanford University School of Medicine.

334 | Dr. Simon Yu

Dr. Yu is certified by the American Board of Internal Medicine, and is a member of the American College of Physicians. He serves on the board of the International College of Integrative Medicine (ICIM), and is active in many integrative medical organizations.

Dr. Yu lectures across the United States and around the world, and has studied Biological Medicine extensively in Europe. Here are some of the experiences that shaped his career.

Dr. Yu attended Dr. Douglas Cook, DDS's "Conference on Energy in Medicine and Dentistry" in Chicago in 1996. Another medical doctor who attended the conference, Dr. Tom Stone, MD, succinctly stated what Dr. Yu felt was his reason for attending: *"To find out how dentists are killing my patients."*

Until this event, Dr. Yu did not realize the magnitude of the relationship between the oral cavity's pathology and patient health. At the conference, Dr. Cook introduced participants to computerized electrodermal screening (CEDS). Skeptical at first, Dr. Yu took a second CEDS course before realizing that the EAV (electroacupuncture according to Voll) tool provides medical doctors or dentists a valuable method for evaluating connections between the teeth and the body.

Dr. Yu began to acquire and test modern, updated digital machines, and developed Acupuncture Meridian Assessment (AMA) to guide detection and treatment of root causes of diseases. Using AMA, he learned how energy meridians and energy fields can transform a medical practice, enabling patients to move beyond lifelong medication of symptoms to restoring health.

In 2001, Dr. Yu's work as an Army Reserve medical officer took him on a mission to Bolivia where he treated 10,000 Andes Indians with parasite medications. He saw this not only resolved parasite problems, but many reported it helped them overcome a range of additional health problems. Dr. Yu's experience treating parasites in Bolivia are noted in chapters 5, 7, 9 and 12 of this book.

Dr. Yu wondered how many of his U.S. patients might be helped by detection and treatment of parasites. He learned to search for evidence of parasite problems using AMA, and saw many of his patients with chronic and unexplained medical conditions respond favorably to antiparasitic medications. Parasite problems are often linked with fungal problems, and he learned to treat these as well.

Dr. Yu's knowledge has been enriched through learning about German Biological Medicine, and attending many annual Medicine Week events and presentations in Baden-Baden, Germany over the years. Walter Sturm, PhD, and his wife Carolyn Winsor, of the Occidental Institute Research Foundation (OIRF) in Canada, organized annual conference tours and presentations with some of the world's most well-respected scientists and biological medicine practitioners. Dr. Yu has been honored to give presentations in connection with Medicine Week over the years, and was invited to give his first international AMA Training, in Germany, in 2019.

Dr. Yu offers Special Training on Acupuncture Meridian Assessment (AMA) for doctors, dentists and prescribing health professionals. He has also organized and hosted ten International Integrative Medicine Conferences. You can order proceedings of the 2017 Conference, Curing the Incurables: Fungal Parasite Dental Conundrum, from Aurora Recording.

He writes a monthly newsletter, and has over 170 articles on his website, and selected videos on his YouTube channel. He thanks his many colleagues who together are shaping the practice and science of medicine and dentistry to address the root causes of cancer and chronic diseases and help restore health.

Acknowledgements

I could not write this book without my wife, Kate's support; I am grateful for her patience and unconditional love. Laura Henze Russell has been instrumental as a writer and editor for helping me organize my many short articles into this book. I also thank Shawn Cornell for his creative cover designs, Scott Forsgren and Kate Sarvasri Hackman, for reviewing the manuscript, Eva Grouling Snider of Russell Media for editing, and Brad Colin for indexing.

I would like to thank the late Harvey Walker, MD, PhD, who introduced me to the world of Integrative Medicine in St. Louis and Walter Sturm, PhD for introducing me to German Biological Medicine. I am also grateful to Douglas Cook, DDS for the introduction to Energy Medicine in the field of Biological Dentistry, and the U.S. Army for providing a unique experience in the Reserve Medical Corps to make this book possible.

I would like to thank the many physicians, dentists and researchers who have given presentations at my ten International Integrative Medicine conferences in St. Louis over the years; some of their contributions are noted in this book. I also want to thank the growing number of doctors, dentists and other prescribing health professionals who attend the Acupuncture Meridian Assessment (AMA) Training sessions I offer twice a year in St. Louis to learn AMA, and consider how to integrate it in their practice.

There are many people who have contributed directly or indirectly for the creation of this book and it is nearly impossible to recognize and acknowledge everyone. I owe many thanks to my family, my staff at Prevention and Healing, my colleagues, my patients and supporters around the world. Together, we face and overcome many knowns and unknowns.

Endnotes

Chapter 2 Develop a Battle Plan against Asymmetric Threats

[1] Daniel L. Davis, "Truth, Lies and Afghanistan," *Armed Forces Journal*, (February 1, 2012), http://armedforcesjournal.com/truth-lies-and-afghanistan/.

[2] David L. Buffaloe, "Defining Asymmetric Warfare," Association of the United States Army, October 1, 2006, https://www.ausa.org/publications/defining-asymmetric-warfare.

[3] Donald Rumsfeld, "NATO Speech: Press Conference US SoD - NATO HQ, Brussels - 6 June 2002," Nato Speeches, June 6, 2002, https://www.nato.int/docu/speech/2002/s020606g.htm.https://www.nato.int/docu/speech/2002/s020606g.htm

[4] Bill Berkrot, "Global prescription drug spend seen at $1.5 trillion in 2021: Report," *Reuters*, December 6, 2016, https://www.reuters.com/article/us-health-pharmaceuticals-spending/global-prescription-drug-spend-seen-at-1-5-trillion-in-2021-report-idUSKBN13V0CB.

[5] Center for Responsive Politics, "Lobbying Spending Database Pharmaceuticals/Health Products, 2017," April 24, 2018, https://www.opensecrets.org/lobby/indusclient.php?id=h04&year=2017. Author's calculation of total. Accessed October 30, 2018.

[6] Barbara Starfield, "Is US Health Really the Best in the World?" *JAMA* 284, no. 4 (July 26, 2000) 483-85, https://doi.org/10.1001/jama.284.4.483.

[7] Gary Null et al., "Death by Medicine," *Journal of Orthomolecular Medicine*, 20, no. 1 (2005): 21-34, accessed November 26, 2018, retrieved from http://orthomolecular.org/library/jom/2005/pdf/2005-v20n01-p021.pdf.

Chapter 3 Accidental Cure and Acupuncture Meridian Assessment

[8] Robert H. Shmerling, "First, Do No Harm," Harvard Health Blog, October 13, 2015, https://www.health.harvard.edu/blog/first-do-no-harm-201510138421.

Chapter 4 Biological Terrain and Biocybernetic Medicine

[9] McMakin, Carolyn, "Dr. McMakin's Publications - Frequency Specific Medicine," accessed November 23, 2018, https://frequencyspecific.com/papers/.

[10] Cleveland Clinic, "Frequency Specific Microcurrent," August 13, 2015, https://my.clevelandclinic.org/health/treatments/15935-frequency-specific-microcurrent.

[11] Daniel Greene, "FDA approved? - Frequency Specific Microcurrent," March 9, 2017, https://frequencyspecific.com/ufaqs/fda-approved/.

Chapter 6 Murder by Dentists: A Mouthful of Forensic Evidence

[12] James S. Woods et al., "Genetic Polymorphisms Affecting Susceptibility to Mercury Neurotoxicity in Children: Summary Findings from the Casa Pia Children's Amalgam Clinical Trial," *Neurotoxicology* 44 (September 2014): 288-302, https://doi.org/10.1016/j.neuro.2014.07.010.

[13] Thomas R. Duplinsky and Domenic V. Cicchetti, "The Health Status of Dentists Exposed to Mercury from mercury Tooth Restorations," *International Journal of Statistics in Medical Research,* 1, no. 1 (2012): 1-15, https://doi.org/10.6000/1929-6029.2012.01.01.01.

[14] Johann Lechner and Volker Von Baehr, "Impact of Endodontically Treated Teeth on Systemic Diseases," *Dentistry* 8, no. 3 (March 31, 2018): 476, accessed November 23, 2018, retrieved from https://www.omicsonline.org/open-access/impact-of-endodontically-treated-teeth-on-systemic-diseases-2161-1122-1000476-100079.html.

[15] William Revak and Susan Revak, "Understanding the Issues with Root Canals, Part One," *OraWellness* (blog), June 18, 2013, accessed November 23, 2018. https://orawellness.com/understanding-the-issues-with-root-canals-part-one/?affiliate=100.

[16] Sim K. Singhrao and Ingar Olsen, "Assessing the Role of Porphyromonas Gingivalis in Periodontitis to Determine a Causative Relationship with Alzheimer's Disease," *Journal of Oral Microbiology* 11, no. 1 (January 29, 2019): 1563405, https://dx.doi.org/10.1080%2F20002297.2018.1563405.

[17] Mark Ide et al, "Periodontitis and Cognitive Decline in Alzheimer's Disease," *PLoS ONE* 11, no. 3 (March 10, 2016): e0151081, https://doi.org/10.1371/journal.pone.0151081.

[18] Keshava Abbayya et al, "Association between Periodontitis and Alzheimer's Disease," *North American Journal of Medical Sciences* 7, no. 6 (June 25, 2015): 241-6, doi:10.4103/1947-2714.159325.

[19] Naoyuki Ishida et al, "Periodontitis induced by bacterial infection exacerbates features of Alzheimer's disease in transgenic mice," *npj Aging and Mechanisms of Disease* 3, no. 1 (November 6, 2017): 15, https://doi.org/10.1038/s41514-017-0015-x .

[20] Bonnie Feldman et al, "The Little Things that Matter – Oral Bacteriophages," Your (Auto)Immunity Connection, (March 22, 2019), https://drbonnie360.com/2019/03/22/the-little-things-that-matter-oral-bacteriophages/.

Chapter 7 Parasites as Masters of Deception

[21] Arabella L. Simpkin and Richard M. Schwartzstein, "Tolerating Uncertainty — The Next Medical Revolution?" *New England Journal of Medicine* 375, no. 18 (November 3, 2016): 1713–15. https://doi.org/10.1056/NEJMp1606402.

[22] Florian H. Pilsczek, "Helminthic Infections Mimicking Malignancy: A Review of Published Case Reports," *The Journal of Infection in Developing Countries,* 4, no. 7 (April 15, 2010): 425-29, https://doi.org/10.3855/jidc.840.

[23] Vassilis Samaras et al, "Chronic Bacterial and Parasitic Infections and Cancer: A Review," *Journal of Infection in Developing Countries,* 4, no. 5 (May 11, 2010): 267-81, https://doi.org/10.3855/jidc.819.

[24] Claudia Gary, "Toxic Hitchhikers: Parasites from War Zones," *Facebook* - Vietnam Veterans of America Northern New Mexico Chapter 996 – Posts (blog), August 21, 2014, https://www.facebook.com/VVAch996/posts/726808357390237.

[25] Jeffrey M. Wilson et al., "Galactose-α-1,3-Galactose: Atypical Food Allergen or Model IgE Hypersensitivity?," *Current Allergy and Asthma Reports,* 17, no. 1 (January 2017):8, https://doi.org/10.1007/s11882-017-0672-7.

[26] Moises Velasquez-Manoff, "What the Mystery of the Tick-Borne Meat Allergy Could Reveal," *The New York Times,* July 24, 2018, https://www.nytimes.com/2018/07/24/magazine/what-the-mystery-of-the-tick-borne-meat-allergy-could-reveal.html.

Chapter 8 Fungal Invaders

[27] Blake T. Aftab et al., "Itraconazole Inhibits Angiogenesis and Tumor Growth in Non-Small Cell Lung Cancer," *Cancer Research* 71, no. 21 (November 1, 2011): 6764-72, https://www.ncbi.nlm.nih.gov/pubmed/21896639.

[28] Blanka Rebacz et al, Identification of griseofulvin as an inhibitor of centrosomal clustering in a phenotype-based screen, *Cancer Research* 67, no. 13 (July 1, 2007): 6342-50. https://doi.org/10.1158/0008-5472.CAN-07-0663.

Chapter 9 Cancer: What Are We Missing?

[29] American Cancer Society, "Cancer Facts & Figures 2018" (Atlanta: American Cancer Society, 2018), p. 2, accessed November 21, 2018, https://www.cancer.org/content/dam/cancer-org/research/cancer-facts-and-statistics/annual-cancer-facts-and-figures/2018/cancer-facts-and-figures-2018.pdf.

[30] National Cancer Institute, "Cancer Statistics," April 27, 2018, accessed November 25, 2018, https://www.cancer.gov/about-cancer/understanding/statistics.

[31] National Cancer Institute, "Annual Report to the Nation 2018: National Cancer Statistics," Surveillance, Epidemiology, and End Results Program (SEER), accessed November 18, 2018, https://seer.cancer.gov/report_to_nation/statistics.html.

[32] Centers for Disease Control and Prevention, "United States Cancer Statistics: Highlights from 2015 Incidence. U.S. Cancer Statistics data brief, no 3." (Centers for Disease Control and Prevention, June 2018), accessed November 18, 2018, https://www.cdc.gov/cancer/uscs/pdf/USCS-DataBrief-No3-June2018-508.pdf.

[33] National Cancer Institute, "Annual Report to the Nation 2018," accessed November 18, 2018, https://seer.cancer.gov/report_to_nation/statistics.html.

[34] American Cancer Society, "Cancer Facts & Figures 2018," op. cit., p. 1.

[35] Andrew C. von Eschenbach, "NCI Sets Goal of Eliminating Suffering and Death Due to Cancer by 2015," *Journal of the National Medical Association* 95, no. 7 (July 2003): 637–39, accessed November 25, 2017, retrieved from https://www.ncbi.nlm.nih.gov/pmc/articles/PMC2594648/.

[36] National Cancer Institute, National Cancer Institute, "NCI Dictionary of Cancer Terms," National Cancer Institute, February 2, 2011, https://www.cancer.gov/publications/dictionaries/cancer-terms.https://www.cancer.gov/publications/dictionaries/cancer-terms.

[37] National Cancer Institute, "What Is Cancer?," National Cancer Institute, September 17, 2007, https://www.cancer.gov/about-cancer/understanding/what-is-cancer. https://www.cancer.gov/about-cancer/understanding/what-is-cancer

[38] National Cancer Institute, "Aflatoxins," March 20, 2015, accessed October 30, 2018, https://www.cancer.gov/about-cancer/causes-prevention/risk/substances/aflatoxins.

[39] National Cancer Institute, "Chronic Inflammation," April 29, 2015, accessed October 30, 2018, https://www.cancer.gov/about-cancer/causes-prevention/risk/chronic-inflammation.

[40] National Cancer Institute, "Infectious Agents," April 29, 2015, accessed October 30, 2018, https://www.cancer.gov/about-cancer/causes-prevention/risk/infectious-agents.

[41] Rossitza Lazova et al., "A Melanoma Brain Metastasis with a Donor-Patient Hybrid Genome following Bone Marrow Transplantation: First Evidence for Fusion in Human Cancer," *PloS One* 8, no. 6 (2013): e66731, https://doi.org/10.1371/journal.pone.0066731.

[42] Bob Weinhold, "Epigenetics: The Science of Change," *Environmental Health Perspectives* 114, no. 3 (March 2006): A160–67, https://dx.doi.org/10.1289%2Fehp.114-a160.https://dx.doi.org/10.1289%2Fehp.114-a160.

[43] Calin Stoicov et al., "Molecular Biology of Gastric Cancer: Helicobacter Infection and Gastric Adenocarcinoma: Bacterial and Host Factors Responsible for Altered Growth Signaling," *Gene* 341 (October 27, 2004): 1–17, https://doi.org/10.1016/j.gene.2004.07.023.https://doi.org/10.1016/j.gene.2004.07.023.

[44] Hisashi Hashimoto et al., "Ivermectin Inactivates the Kinase PAK1 and Blocks the PAK1-Dependent Growth of Human Ovarian Cancer and NF2 Tumor Cell Lines," *Drug Discoveries & Therapeutics* 3, no. 6 (December 2009): 243-46. Accessed November 25, 2018, retrieved from http://www.ddtjournal.com/getabstract.php?id=264.

[45] Rafal Bartoszewski et al., "The Unfolded Protein Response (UPR)-Activated Transcription Factor X-Box-Binding Protein 1 (XBP1) Induces MicroRNA-346 Expression That Targets the Human Antigen Peptide Transporter 1 (TAP1) mRNA and Governs Immune Regulatory Genes," *The Journal of Biological Chemistry*, 286, no. 48 (December 2, 2011): 41862–70, https://doi.org/10.1074/jbc.M111.304956.

[46] Sumaiya Sharmeen et al., "The Antiparasitic Agent Ivermectin Induces Chloride-Dependent Membrane Hyperpolarization and Cell Death in Leukemia Cells," *Blood* 116, no. 18 (November 4, 2010): 3593-3603. https://doi.org/10.1182/blood-2010-01-262675.

[47] Zhen Hua Wu et al, "Praziquantel Synergistically Enhances Paclitaxel Efficacy to Inhibit Cancer Cell Growth," *PLOS ONE* 7, no. 12 (December 12, 2012): e51721, https://doi.org/10.1371/journal.pone.0051721.

[48] Jing-Xuan Pan, Ke Ding, and Cheng-Yan Wang, "Niclosamide, an Old Antihelminthic Agent, Demonstrates Antitumor Activity by Blocking Multiple Signaling Pathways of Cancer Stem Cells," *Chinese Journal of Cancer* 31, no. 4 (April 2012): 178–84, https://doi.org/10.5732/cjc.011.10290 .

[49] Rebecca Lamb et al, "Antibiotics that target mitochondria effectively eradicate cancer stem cells, across multiple tumor types: treating cancer like an infectious disease," *Oncotarget* 6, no. 7 (March 10, 2015): 4569-84, https://doi.org/10.18632/oncotarget.3174.

Chapter 10 Lyme and Persistent Lyme

[50] Patient Centered Care Advocacy Group, "Lyme Bacteria Hides Inside Parasitic Worms, Causing Chronic Brain Diseases," Washington, DC: PR Newswire, May 19, 2016, accessed October 30, 2018, https://www.prnewswire.com/news-releases/lyme-bacteria-hides-inside-parasitic-worms-causing-chronic-brain-diseases-300270742.html.

[51] Scott Forsgren and Dietrich Klinghardt, "Kryptopyrroluria 2017: A Major Piece of the Puzzle in Overcoming Chronic Lyme Disease," *Townsend Letter*, July 2017, http://www.townsendletter.com/July2017/krypto0717.html.

Chapter 11 Extraordinary Patients and Unexplained Diseases

[52] National Center for Chronic Disease Prevention and Health Promotion, "About Chronic Disease | Chronic Disease Prevention and Health Promotion | CDC," October 25, 2018, accessed October 30, 2018, https://www.cdc.gov/chronicdisease/about/index.htm.

[53] National Center for Chronic Disease Prevention and Health Promotion, "Health and Economic Costs of Chronic Disease | CDC," October 25, 2018, accessed October 30, 2018, https://www.cdc.gov/chronicdisease/about/costs/index.htm.

[54] T.R. Reid, "How We Spend $3,400,000,000,000," *The Atlantic*, June 15, 2017, accessed October 30, 2018, https://www.theatlantic.com/health/archive/2017/06/how-we-spend-3400000000000/530355/.

[55] Yasmeen Abutaleb, "U.S. Healthcare Spending to Climb 5.3 Percent in 2018: Agency," *Reuters*, February 14, 2018, accessed October 30, 2018, https://www.reuters.com/article/us-usa-healthcare-spending/u-s-healthcare-spending-to-climb-5-3-percent-in-2018-agency-idUSKCN1FY2ZD.

[56] David Blumenthal, "Drop in Life Expectancy an 'Indictment of the American Health Care System'," *STAT*, January 4, 2018, accessed October 30, 2018, https://www.statnews.com/2018/01/04/life-expectancy-us-health-care/.

[57] ProCon, "35 FDA-Approved Prescription Drugs Later Pulled from the Market," January 30, 2014, accessed January 30, 2019, https://prescriptiondrugs.procon.org/view.resource.php?resourceID=005528.

[58] US Food & Drug Administration, Center for Drug Evaluation & Research, Drug Recalls, April 12, 2019, accessed April 12, 2019, https://www.fda.gov/Drugs/DrugSafety/DrugRecalls/default.htm.

[59] Ibid, Drug Safety and Availability - Drug Safety Communications, April 9, 2019, accessed April 12, 2019, https://www.fda.gov/Drugs/DrugSafety/ucm199082.htm.

[60] Laura Henze Russell, "Congress needs to turn its attention to medical device safety," StatNews, December 21, 2016, accessed January 30, 2019, https://www.statnews.com/2016/12/21/medical-devices-safety-congress/.

[61] US Food & Drug Administration, Center for Devices and Radiological Health, Medical Device Bans, September 25, 2018, accessed January 30, 2019, https://www.fda.gov/MedicalDevices/Safety/MedicalDeviceBans/default.htm.

[62] Ibid, Medical Device Safety, January 29, 2019, accessed January 30, 2019, https://www.fda.gov/MedicalDevices/Safety/default.htm.

[63] US Food & Drug Administration, Office of the Commissioner, MedWatch: The FDA Safety Information and Adverse Event Reporting Program, January 29, 2019, accessed January 30, 2019, https://www.fda.gov/Safety/MedWatch/default.htm.

List of Dr. Yu's Articles

*All of Dr. Simon Yu's monthly articles are posted on his website,
www.preventionandhealing.com, on the articles/blog page.*

In-Depth Articles

Recommended Reading

Becker, Robert, and Gary Selden. *The Body Electric: Electromagnetism and The Foundation Of Life*. New York: William Morrow Paperbacks, 1998.

Breiner, Mark A. *Whole-Body Dentistry: A Complete Guide to Understanding the Impact of Dentistry on Total Health*. Fairfield, CT: Quantum Health Press, 2011.

Cook, Douglas L. *Rescued By My Dentist: New Solutions to a Health Crisis*. BC, Canada: Trafford Publishing, 2009.

Dach, Jeffrey L. *Heart Book: How to Keep Your Heart Healthy*. First edition. Davie, FL: Medical Muse Press, 2018.

Gerber, Richard. *A Practical Guide to Vibrational Medicine: Energy Healing and Spiritual Transformation*. New York & London: William Morrow Paperbacks, 2001.

———. *Vibrational Medicine: The #1 Handbook of Subtle-Energy Therapies*. Rochester, VT: Bear & Company, 2001.

Horowitz, Richard. *How Can I Get Better? An Action Plan for Treating Resistant Lyme & Chronic Disease*. New York: St. Martin's Griffin, 2017.

———. *Why Can't I Get Better? Solving the Mystery of Lyme and Chronic Disease*. New York: St. Martin's Press, 2013.

Huggins, Hal A., and Thomas E. Levy. *Uninformed Consent: The Hidden Dangers in Dental Care*. Charlottesville, VA: Hampton Roads Publishing, 1999.

Kaufmann, Doug A. *The Germ That Causes Cancer*. Rockwall, TX: Mediatrition, 2002.

Lane, Nick. *The Vital Question: Energy, Evolution, and the Origins of Complex Life*. New York: Norton & Company, 2016.

Levy, Thomas E. *Hidden Epidemic: Silent Oral Infections Cause Most Heart Attacks and Breast Cancers*. Henderson, Nevada: MedFox Publishing, 2017.

McFadden, Johnjoe, and Jim Al-Khalili. *Life on the Edge: The Coming of Age of Quantum Biology*. NY: Broadway Books, 2016.

McMakin, Carolyn. *The Resonance Effect: How Frequency Specific Microcurrent Is Changing Medicine*. Berkeley, CA: North Atlantic Books, 2017.

Meinig, George E. *Root Canal Cover Up*. 9th Printing edition. Lemon Grove, CA: Price Pottenger Nutrition, 2008.

Meyer, Nicholas J. *The Holistic Dental Matrix: How Teeth Can Control Your Health & Well-Being*. Scottsdale: Millennium, 2016.

Mukherjee, Siddhartha. *The Emperor of All Maladies: A Biography of Cancer*. New York: Scribner, 2010.

Nathan, Neil. *Toxic: Heal Your Body from Mold Toxicity, Lyme Disease, Multiple Chemical Sensitivities, and Chronic Environmental Illness*. Las Vegas: Victory Belt Publishing, 2018.

Oschman, James L. *Energy Medicine: The Scientific Basis*. Edinburgh: Churchill Livingstone, 2015.

Pollack, Gerald H. *The Fourth Phase of Water: Beyond Solid, Liquid, and Vapor*. Seattle, WA: Ebner & Sons, 2013.

Seyfried, Thomas. *Cancer as a Metabolic Disease: On the Origin, Management, and Prevention of Cancer*. Hoboken: Wiley, 2012.

Shoemaker, Ritchie C. *Surviving Mold: Life in the Era of Dangerous Buildings*. Baltimore: Otter Bay Books, 2010.

Swanson, Claude. *Life Force, the Scientific Basis: Volume 2 of the Synchronized Universe*. Tucson, AZ: Poseidia Press, 2011.

————. *Synchronized Universe: New Science of the Paranormal.* Tucson, AZ: Poseidia Press, 2003.

Tennant, Jerry L. *Healing Is Voltage: The Handbook, 3rd Edition.* CreateSpace Independent Publishing Platform, 2010.

Trowbridge, John P., and Morton Walker. *The Yeast Syndrome: How to Help Your Doctor Identify & Treat the Real Cause of Your Yeast-Related Illness.* Toronto & NY: Bantam, 1986.

Yu, Simon. *Accidental Cure: Extraordinary Medicine for Extraordinary Patients.* St. Louis: Prevention and Healing, 2010.

Bibliography

Abutaleb, Yasmeen. "U.S. Healthcare Spending to Climb 5.3 Percent in 2018: Agency." *Reuters*, February 14, 2018. https://www.reuters.com/article/us-usa-healthcare-spending-idUSKCN1FY2ZD.

Abbayya, Keshava, Nagraj Y Puthanakar, Sanjay Naduwinmani, and Y S Chidambar. "Association between Periodontitis and Alzheimer's Disease." *North American Journal of Medical Sciences* 7, no. 6 (June 2015): 241–46. https://doi.org/10.4103/1947-2714.159325.

Aftab, Blake T., Irina Dobromilskaya, Jun O. Liu, and Charles M. Rudin. "Itraconazole Inhibits Angiogenesis and Tumor Growth in Non-Small Cell Lung Cancer." *Cancer Research* 71, no. 21 (November 1, 2011): 6764–72. https://doi.org/10.1158/0008-5472.CAN-11-0691.

American Cancer Society. "Cancer Facts & Figures 2018." Atlanta: American Cancer Society, 2018. https://www.cancer.org/content/dam/cancer-org/research/cancer-facts-and-statistics/annual-cancer-facts-and-figures/2018/cancer-facts-and-figures-2018.pdf

Bartoszewski, Rafal, Joseph W. Brewer, Andras Rab, David K. Crossman, Sylwia Bartoszewska, Niren Kapoor, Cathy Fuller, James F. Collawn, and Zsuzsa Bebok. "The Unfolded Protein Response (UPR)-Activated Transcription Factor X-Box-Binding Protein 1 (XBP1) Induces MicroRNA-346 Expression That Targets the Human Antigen Peptide Transporter 1 (TAP1) MRNA and Governs Immune Regulatory Genes." *The Journal of Biological Chemistry* 286, no. 48 (December 2, 2011): 41862–70. https://doi.org/10.1074/jbc.M111.304956.

Berkrot, Bill. "Global Prescription Drug Spend Seen at $1.5 Trillion in 2021: Report." *Reuters* (December 6, 2016). https://www.reuters.com/article/us-health-pharmaceuticals-spending-idUSKBN13V0CB.

Blumenthal, David. "Drop in Life Expectancy an 'Indictment of the American Health Care System.'" STAT, January 4, 2018. https://www.statnews.com/2018/01/04/life-expectancy-us-health-care/.

Buffaloe, David L. "Defining Asymmetric Warfare." Association of the United States Army, October 1, 2006. https://www.ausa.org/publications/defining-asymmetric-warfare.

Center for Responsive Politics. "Lobbying Spending Database Pharmaceuticals/Health Products, 2017 | OpenSecrets," April 24, 2018. https://www.opensecrets.org/lobby/indusclient.php?id=h04&year=2017.

Centers for Disease Control and Prevention. "United States Cancer Statistics: Highlights from 2015 Incidence. U.S. Cancer Statistics Data Brief, No 3." Centers for Disease Control and Prevention, June 2018. https://www.cdc.gov/cancer/uscs/pdf/USCS-DataBrief-No3-June2018-508.pdf

Cleveland Clinic. "Frequency-Specific Microcurrent," August 13, 2015. https://my.clevelandclinic.org/health/treatments/15935-frequency-specific-microcurrent.

Dach, Jeffrey L. *Heart Book: How to Keep Your Heart Healthy.* First edition. Davie, FL: Medical Muse Press, 2018. https://www.amazon.com/Heart-Book-Keep-Your-Healthy/dp/1732421005/

Davis, Daniel L. "Truth, Lies and Afghanistan." *Armed Forces Journal* Feb. 1, 2012 (February 1, 2012). http://armedforcesjournal.com/truth-lies-and-afghanistan/.

Duplinsky, Thomas R., and Domenic V. Cicchetti. "The Health Status of Dentists Exposed to Mercury from Silver Amalgam Tooth Restorations." *International Journal of Statistics in Medical Research* 1, no. 1 (2012): 1–15. https://doi.org/10.6000/1929-6029.2012.01.01.01.

Eschenbach, Andrew C. von. "NCI Sets Goal of Eliminating Suffering and Death Due to Cancer by 2015." *Journal of the National Medical Association* 95, no. 7 (July 2003): 637–39. Retrieved from https://www.ncbi.nlm.nih.gov/pmc/articles/PMC2594648/.

Feldman, Bonnie. "The Little Things That Matter — Oral Bacteriophages – DrBonnie360 Presents." Your (Auto)Immunity Connection, March 22, 2019. https://drbonnie360.com/2019/03/22/the-little-things-that-matter-oral-bacteriophages/.

Forsgren, Scott. "Cavitation Journey." BetterHealthGuy.com - A Site Dedicated to Lyme Disease and Mold Illness, December 21, 2013, updated February 26, 2018. https://www.betterhealthguy.com/cavitation.

Forsgren, Scott. "Simon Who? Yes, That's Right. Simon Yu MD." BetterHealthGuy.com - A Site Dedicated to Lyme Disease and Mold Illness. September 12, 2013, updated March 14, 2019. https://www.betterhealthguy.com/yu.

Forsgren, Scott and Dietrich Klinghardt. "Kryptopyrroluria 2017: A Major Piece of the Puzzle in Overcoming Chronic Lyme Disease." *Townsend Letter* (July 2017). http://www.townsendletter.com/July2017/krypto0717.html.

Gary, Claudia. "Toxic Hitchhikers: Parasites from War Zones." Facebook - Vietnam Veterans of America Northern New Mexico Chapter 996 - Posts, August 21, 2014. https://www.facebook.com/VVAch996/posts/726808357390237.

Greene, Daniel. "FDA Approved? - Frequency Specific Microcurrent," March 9, 2017. https://frequencyspecific.com/ufaqs/fda-approved/.

Hashimoto, H., S. M. Messerli, T. Sudo, and H. Maruta. "Ivermectin Inactivates the Kinase PAK1 and Blocks the PAK1-Dependent Growth of Human Ovarian Cancer and NF2 Tumor Cell Lines." *Drug Discoveries & Therapeutics* 3, no. 6 (December 2009): 243–46. Retrieved from http://www.ddtjournal.com/getabstract.php?id=264.

Ide, Mark, Marina Harris, Annette Stevens, Rebecca Sussams, Viv Hopkins, David Culliford, et al. "Periodontitis and Cognitive Decline in Alzheimer's Disease." *PLoS ONE* 11, no. 3 (March 10, 2016): e0151081. https://doi.org/10.1371/journal.pone.0151081.

Ishida, Naoyuki, Yuichi Ishihara, Kazuto Ishida, Hiroyuki Tada, Yoshiko Funaki-Kato, Makoto Hagiwara, Taslima Ferdous, et al. "Periodontitis Induced by Bacterial Infection Exacerbates Features of Alzheimer's Disease in Transgenic Mice." *Npj Aging and Mechanisms of Disease* 3, no. 1 (November 6, 2017): 15. https://doi.org/10.1038/s41514-017-0015-x.

Lamb, Rebecca, Bela Ozsvari, Camilla L. Lisanti, Herbert B. Tanowitz, Anthony Howell, Ubaldo E. Martinez-Outschoorn, Federica Sotgia, and Michael P. Lisanti. "Antibiotics That Target Mitochondria Effectively Eradicate Cancer Stem Cells, across Multiple Tumor Types: Treating Cancer like an Infectious Disease." *Oncotarget* 6, no. 7 (March 10, 2015): 4569–84. https://doi.org/10.18632/oncotarget.3174.

Lazova, Rossitza, Greggory S. Laberge, Eric Duvall, Nicole Spoelstra, Vincent Klump, Mario Sznol, Dennis Cooper, Richard A. Spritz, Joseph T. Chang, and John M. Pawelek. "A Melanoma Brain Metastasis with a Donor-Patient Hybrid Genome Following Bone Marrow Transplantation: First Evidence for Fusion in Human Cancer." *PloS One* 8, no. 6 (2013): e66731. https://doi.org/10.1371/journal.pone.0066731.

Lechner, Johann, and Volker Von Baehr. "Impact of Endodontically Treated Teeth on Systemic Diseases." *Dentistry* 8, no. 3 (March 31, 2018): 476. Retrieved from https://www.omicsonline.org/open-access/impact-of-endodontically-treated-teeth-on-systemic-diseases-2161-1122-1000476-100079.html.

Levy, Thomas E, *Hidden Epidemic: Silent Oral Infections Cause Most Heart Attacks and Breast Cancers.* Henderson, NV: Medfox Publishing, 2017. https://www.amazon.com/Hidden-Epidemic-Infections-Attacks-Cancers/dp/0983772878.

McMakin, Carolyn. *The Resonance Effect: How Frequency Specific Microcurrent Is Changing Medicine.* Berkeley, CA: North Atlantic Books, 2017. https://www.amazon.com/Resonance-Effect-Frequency-Specific-Microcurrent/dp/1623171105.

McMakin, Carolyn. "Dr. McMakin's Publications - Frequency Specific Medicine." Accessed November 23, 2018. https://frequencyspecific.com/papers/.

Nathan, Neil. *Toxic: Heal Your Body from Mold Toxicity, Lyme Disease, Multiple Chemical Sensitivities, and Chronic Environmental Illness.* Las Vegas, NV: Victory Belt Publishing, 2018. https://www.amazon.com/Toxic-Toxicity-Multiple-Sensitivities-Environmental-ebook/dp/B07H72N9RH.

National Cancer Institute. "Aflatoxins." Article. National Cancer Institute, March 20, 2015. https://www.cancer.gov/about-cancer/causes-prevention/risk/substances/aflatoxins.

———. "Annual Report to the Nation 2018: National Cancer Statistics." Surveillance, Epidemiology, and End Results Program (SEER). https://seer.cancer.gov/report_to_nation/statistics.html.

———. "Cancer Statistics." Article. National Cancer Institute, April 27, 2018. https://www.cancer.gov/about-cancer/understanding/statistics.

———. "Chronic Inflammation." Article. National Cancer Institute, April 29, 2015. https://www.cancer.gov/about-cancer/causes-prevention/risk/chronic-inflammation.

———. "Infectious Agents." Article. National Cancer Institute, April 29, 2015. https://www.cancer.gov/about-cancer/causes-prevention/risk/infectious-agents.

———. "What Is Cancer?" Article. National Cancer Institute, September 17, 2007. https://www.cancer.gov/about-cancer/understanding/what-is-cancer.

———. "NCI Dictionary of Cancer Terms." National Cancer Institute, February 2, 2011. https://www.cancer.gov/publications/dictionaries/cancer-terms.

National Center for Chronic Disease Prevention and Health Promotion. "About Chronic Disease | Chronic Disease Prevention and Health Promotion | CDC," October 25, 2018. https://www.cdc.gov/chronicdisease/about/index.htm.

———. "Health and Economic Costs of Chronic Disease | CDC," October 25, 2018. https://www.cdc.gov/chronicdisease/about/costs/index.htm.

Null, Gary, Carolyn Dean, Martin Feldman, and Debora Rasio. "Death by Medicine." *Journal of Orthomolecular Medicine* 20, no. 1 (2005): 21–34. Retrieved from http://www.orthomolecular.org/library/jom/2005/pdf/2005-v20n01-p021.pdf.

Pan, Jing-Xuan, Ke Ding, and Cheng-Yan Wang. "Niclosamide, an Old Antihelminthic Agent, Demonstrates Antitumor Activity by Blocking Multiple Signaling Pathways of Cancer Stem Cells." *Chinese Journal of Cancer* 31, no. 4 (April 2012): 178–84. https://doi.org/10.5732/cjc.011.10290

Patient Centered Care Advocacy Group. "Lyme Bacteria Hides Inside Parasitic Worms, Causing Chronic Brain Diseases," May 19, 2016. https://www.prnewswire.com/news-releases.detail.html//content/prnewswire/us/en/news-releases.detail.html/lyme-bacteria-hides-inside-parasitic-worms-causing-chronic-brain-diseases-300270742.html.html.

Pilsczek, Florian H. "Helminthic Infections Mimicking Malignancy: A Review of Published Case Reports." *The Journal of Infection in Developing Countries* 4, no. 07 (April 15, 2010): 425–29. https://doi.org/10.3855/jidc.840.

ProCon.org. "35 FDA-Approved Prescription Drugs Later Pulled from the Market - Prescription Drug Ads." ProCon.org, January 30, 2014. https://prescriptiondrugs.procon.org/view.resource.php?resourceID=005528.

Rebacz, Blanka, Thomas O. Larsen, Mads H. Clausen, Mads H. Rønnest, Harald Löffler, Anthony D. Ho, and Alwin Krämer. "Identification of Griseofulvin as an Inhibitor of Centrosomal Clustering in a Phenotype-Based Screen." *Cancer Research* 67, no. 13 (July 1, 2007): 6342–50. https://doi.org/10.1158/0008-5472.CAN-07-0663.

Reid, T. R. "How We Spend $3,400,000,000,000." The Atlantic, June 15, 2017. https://www.theatlantic.com/health/archive/2017/06/how-we-spend-3400000000000/530355/.

Revak, William, and Susan Revak. "Understanding the Issues with Root Canals, Part One." *OraWellness* (blog), June 18, 2013. https://orawellness.com/understanding-the-issues-with-root-canals-part-one/.

Russell, Laura Henze. "Congress Needs to Turn Its Attention to Medical Device Safety." *StatNews*, December 21, 2016. https://www.statnews.com/2016/12/21/medical-devices-safety-congress/.

Rumsfeld, Donald. "NATO Speech: Press Conference US SoD - NATO HQ, Brussels - 6 June 2002." Nato Speeches, June 6, 2002. https://www.nato.int/docu/speech/2002/s020606g.htm.

Samaras, Vassilis, Petros I. Rafailidis, Eleni G. Mourtzoukou, George Peppas, and Matthew E. Falagas. "Chronic Bacterial and Parasitic Infections and Cancer: A Review." *The Journal of Infection in Developing Countries* 4, no. 05 (May 11, 2010): 267–81. https://doi.org/10.3855/jidc.819.

Sharmeen, Sumaiya, Marko Skrtic, Mahadeo A. Sukhai, Rose Hurren, Marcela Gronda, Xiaoming Wang, Sonali B. Fonseca, et al. "The Antiparasitic Agent Ivermectin Induces Chloride-Dependent Membrane Hyperpolarization and Cell Death in Leukemia Cells." *Blood* 116, no. 18 (November 4, 2010): 3593–3603. https://doi.org/10.1182/blood-2010-01-262675.

Shmerling, MD, Robert H. "First, Do No Harm." Harvard Health Blog, October 13, 2015. https://www.health.harvard.edu/blog/first-do-no-harm-201510138421.

Simpkin, Arabella L., and Richard M. Schwartzstein. "Tolerating Uncertainty — The Next Medical Revolution?" *New England Journal of Medicine* 375, no. 18 (November 3, 2016): 1713–15. https://doi.org/10.1056/NEJMp1606402.

Singhrao, Sim K., and Ingar Olsen. "Assessing the Role of Porphyromonas Gingivalis in Periodontitis to Determine a Causative Relationship with Alzheimer's Disease." *Journal of Oral Microbiology* 11, no. 1 (January 1, 2019): 1563405. https://doi.org/10.1080/20002297.2018.1563405.

Starfield, Barbara. "Is US Health Really the Best in the World?" *JAMA* 284, no. 4 (July 26, 2000): 483–85. https://doi.org/10.1001/jama.284.4.483.

Stoicov, Calin, Reza Saffari, Xun Cai, Chhaya Hasyagar, and JeanMarie Houghton. "Molecular Biology of Gastric Cancer: Helicobacter Infection and Gastric Adenocarcinoma: Bacterial and Host Factors Responsible for Altered Growth Signaling." *Gene* 341 (October 27, 2004): 1–17. https://doi.org/10.1016/j.gene.2004.07.023.

US Food & Drug Administration, Center for Devices and Radiological Health. "Medical Device Safety." WebContent, April 11, 2019. https://www.fda.gov/MedicalDevices/Safety/default.htm.

———, Center for Devices and Radiological Health. "Medical Device Bans." WebContent. Accessed April 12, 2019. https://www.fda.gov/MedicalDevices/Safety/MedicalDeviceBans/default.htm.

———, Center for Drug Evaluation and Research. "Drug Recalls." WebContent, April 12, 2019. https://www.fda.gov/Drugs/DrugSafety/DrugRecalls/default.htm.

———, Center for Drug Evaluation and Research. "Drug Safety and Availability - Drug Safety Communications." WebContent, April 12, 2019. https://www.fda.gov/Drugs/DrugSafety/ucm199082.htm.

———, Office of the Commissioner. "MedWatch: The FDA Safety Information and Adverse Event Reporting Program." WebContent. Accessed April 12, 2019. https://www.fda.gov/Safety/MedWatch/default.htm.

Velasquez-Manoff, Moises. "What the Mystery of the Tick-Borne Meat Allergy Could Reveal - The New York Times," July 24, 2018. https://www.nytimes.com/2018/07/24/magazine/what-the-mystery-of-the-tick-borne-meat-allergy-could-reveal.html.

Weinhold, Bob. "Epigenetics: The Science of Change." *Environmental Health Perspectives* 114, no. 3 (March 2006): A160–67. https://dx.doi.org/10.1289%2Fehp.114-a160.

Wilson, Jeffrey M., Alexander J. Schuyler, Nikhila Schroeder, and Thomas A. E. Platts-Mills. "Galactose-α-1,3-Galactose: Atypical Food Allergen or Model IgE Hypersensitivity?" *Current Allergy and Asthma Reports* 17, no. 1 (January 2017): 8. https://doi.org/10.1007/s11882-017-0672-7.

Woods, James S., Nicholas J. Heyer, Joan E. Russo, Michael D. Martin, and Federico M. Farin. "Genetic Polymorphisms Affecting Susceptibility to Mercury Neurotoxicity in Children: Summary Findings from the Casa Pia Children's Amalgam Clinical Trial." *Neurotoxicology* 44 (September 2014): 288–302. https://doi.org/10.1016/j.neuro.2014.07.010.

Wu, Zhen Hua, Ming-ke Lu, Long Yu Hu, and Xiaotong Li. "Praziquantel Synergistically Enhances Paclitaxel Efficacy to Inhibit Cancer Cell Growth." *PLOS ONE* 7, no. 12 (December 12, 2012). https://doi.org/10.1371/journal.pone.0051721.

Yu, Simon. Accidental Cure: Extraordinary Medicine for Extraordinary Patients. St. Louis, MO: Prevention and Healing, Inc., 2010. https://www.amazon.com/Accidental-Cure-Extraordinary-Medicine-Patients/dp/0979734266.

INDEX

C

Cadmium, 56, 329
Cancer
breast cancer, 60–61
carcinoma, 195
causes of, 197
definition of, 194–196
leukemia, 195
liver cancer, 63, 154
lung cancer, 60–61
lymphoma, 195
multiple myeloma, 195
nose and throat cancer, 198
sarcoma, 195
skin cancer, 190, 194, 198
symptoms of, 67
war on, 35, 38, 48–66, 192, 194, 227
Cancer of Left Leg, 207–212. *See also Cancer; causes of*
Candida albicans, 186
Canker sores, 157
Cantin, Elaine, 234
Cardiomyopathy, 157, 240, 251
Cardiovascular disease, 122, 163
Carlin, George, 64
Celiac disease, 157
Centers for Disease Control and Prevention (CDC), 153, 169, 189–190, 195, 231, 240, 248, 250, 254
Central Nervous System, 104, 196, 269
Chandler, David G., 52
Chelation Therapy, 31, 55, 82, 210, 269, 275–276, 299, 329
Chemotherapy, 29, 34–36, 39–41, 54, 62–67, 70, 85, 161, 192–193, 199, 202–208, 212, 226–229, 233, 276, 325–326
Cheryl's Story, 38
Children's Amalgam Trial, 133
Chilton, Kevin P., 53
Chlamydia, 153, 179
Cholestyramine, 183
Chronic bacterial, 153
Chronic Diseases, 26–27, 30, 33–34, 42, 45–46, 58, 68, 115, 119, 126–127, 183, 200, 225, 254–255, 259, 332
Chronic Fatigue, 48, 75, 101–102, 110, 135–136, 148, 152, 163, 240, 244, 251, 253, 258–259, 264–265, 271–275, 280, 306, 320. *See also Chronic Fatigue Syndrome (CFS/CFIDS)*
Chronic fatigue and immune dysfunction syndrome (CFIDS), 136, 275, 320

Malarial plasmodium parasite, 176
Malnutrition, 56
McFadden, Johnjoe, 99
McMakin, Carolyn, 96, 98–99
Mebendazole, 110, 231, 280, 282–283, 286–287, 290–293
Medical Devices, 57, 142, 256–258
Medically unexplained symptoms (MUS), 29, 84, 115, 227–230, 253, 259, 263–265, 308
Meinig, George, 134, 272
Memory loss, 158
Mental illness, 177–179
Mercury, 31, 40, 43, 56, 89, 102, 107, 119–123, 126, 132–134, 137–138, 142–147, 208, 215–216, 220, 257, 265, 269, 298–299, 329–330
Meridians
Allergy, 102, 114, 207–208
Bladder, 101, 108, 283
Dental (lymph), 102, 138, 206
Gallbladder, 101–105, 173, 206, 283
Heart, 101, 106–109, 283
Kidney, 101, 283
Large Intestine (LI), 101–102, 110–113,
173, 206, 283
Liver, 101, 104, 173, 206, 283
Lung, 101, 110–111
Lymph (dental), 102, 283
Pancreas (spleen), 283
Pericardium, 101, 104, 283
Prostate (bladder), 107–108, 283
Small Intestine (SI), 101–102, 173, 283
Spleen (pancreas), 101, 111, 283
Stomach, 101, 111, 206, 283
Triple Warmer, 101, 104, 160, 283
Uterus (bladder), 283
Merkel Cell polyomavirus (MCPyV), 198
Metabolic, 30, 33, 42, 56, 92, 201, 221, 231–232, 234–238
Metabolic disease, 201, 221, 232, 236, 238
Metabolism, 30, 32, 55, 119, 151, 202, 232–236, 285, 288–289, 311
Metastasis, 36, 38, 66, 188, 196, 200, 206, 210, 213, 223
Metronidazole (Flagyl), 288
Meyer, Nicholas J., 121
Microbiome, 30, 32–34, 47, 57, 119, 151, 176–177

CPSIA information can be obtained
at www.ICGtesting.com
Printed in the USA
FFHW020133270619
53235631-58909FF